GUIDING CANCER CONTROL

A Path to Transformation

Michael M. E. Johns, Guru Madhavan,
Francis K. Amankwah, and Sharyl J. Nass, *Editors*

Committee on a National Strategy for Cancer Control
in the United States

Board on Health Care Services

Health and Medicine Division

A Consensus Study Report of

The National Academies of
SCIENCES · ENGINEERING · MEDICINE

THE NATIONAL ACADEMIES PRESS
Washington, DC
www.nap.edu

THE NATIONAL ACADEMIES PRESS 500 Fifth Street, NW Washington, DC 20001

This activity was supported by grants from the American Cancer Society, the Centers for Disease Control and Prevention, and the National Cancer Institute of the National Institutes of Health. Any opinions, findings, conclusions, or recommendations expressed in this publication do not necessarily reflect the views of any organization that provided support for the project.

International Standard Book Number-13: 978-0-309-49231-7
International Standard Book Number-10: 0-309-49231-9
Digital Object Identifier: https://doi.org/10.17226/25438
Library of Congress Control Number: 2019944355

Additional copies of this publication are available from the National Academies Press, 500 Fifth Street, NW, Keck 360, Washington, DC 20001; (800) 624-6242 or (202) 334-3313; www.nap.edu.

Printed in the United States of America

Suggested citation: National Academies of Sciences, Engineering, and Medicine. 2019. *Guiding cancer control: A path to transformation*. Washington, DC: The National Academies Press. doi: https://doi.org/10.17226/25438.

The National Academies of

SCIENCES • ENGINEERING • MEDICINE

The **National Academy of Sciences** was established in 1863 by an Act of Congress, signed by President Lincoln, as a private, nongovernmental institution to advise the nation on issues related to science and technology. Members are elected by their peers for outstanding contributions to research. Dr. Marcia McNutt is president.

The **National Academy of Engineering** was established in 1964 under the charter of the National Academy of Sciences to bring the practices of engineering to advising the nation. Members are elected by their peers for extraordinary contributions to engineering. Dr. C. D. Mote, Jr., is president.

The **National Academy of Medicine** (formerly the Institute of Medicine) was established in 1970 under the charter of the National Academy of Sciences to advise the nation on medical and health issues. Members are elected by their peers for distinguished contributions to medicine and health. Dr. Victor J. Dzau is president.

The three Academies work together as the **National Academies of Sciences, Engineering, and Medicine** to provide independent, objective analysis and advice to the nation and conduct other activities to solve complex problems and inform public policy decisions. The National Academies also encourage education and research, recognize outstanding contributions to knowledge, and increase public understanding in matters of science, engineering, and medicine.

Learn more about the National Academies of Sciences, Engineering, and Medicine at **www.nationalacademies.org**.

The National Academies of
SCIENCES • ENGINEERING • MEDICINE

COMMITTEE ON A NATIONAL STRATEGY FOR CANCER CONTROL IN THE UNITED STATES

MICHAEL M. E. JOHNS (*Chair*), Chancellor Emeritus and Professor of Medicine and Public Health, Emory University; President and Chief Executive Officer Emeritus, Emory Healthcare

KATRINA ARMSTRONG, Jackson Professor of Clinical Medicine, Harvard Medical School; Chair, Department of Medicine, and Physician-in-Chief, Massachusetts General Hospital

SMITA BHATIA, Gay and Bew White Endowed Chair in Pediatric Oncology; Director, Institute for Cancer Outcomes and Survivorship; University of Alabama School of Medicine

BETTY FERRELL, Director and Professor, Division of Nursing Research and Education, City of Hope National Medical Center

JONATHAN FIELDING, Distinguished Professor of Health Policy and Management and Pediatrics, University of California, Los Angeles; Former Los Angeles County Director of Public Health

BEVERLY ASHLEIGH GUADAGNOLO, Professor of Radiation Oncology and Health Services Research; Section Chief, Sarcoma/ Melanoma Radiation Oncology; Associate Director of Physicians Referral Service, The University of Texas MD Anderson Cancer Center

JOSEPH LIPSCOMB, Georgia Cancer Coalition Distinguished Cancer Scholar and Professor of Health Policy and Management, Emory University

MARÍA ELENA MARTÍNEZ, Sam M. Walton Endowed Chair for Cancer Research and Professor of Family and Preventive Medicine, University of California, San Diego

MARY McCABE, Consultant in Cancer Survivorship, and Former Clinical Director, Cancer Survivorship Center, Memorial Sloan Kettering Cancer Center

LEAH MERCHANT, Section Supervisor, Montana Cancer Control Programs, Montana Department of Public Health and Human Services

JEWEL MULLEN, Associate Dean for Health Equity and Associate Professor of Population Health and Internal Medicine, The University of Texas at Austin Dell Medical School

ELECTRA PASKETT, Marion N. Rowley Professor of Cancer Research, The Ohio State University

GEORGE POSTE, Regents' Professor and Del E. Webb Chair of Health Innovation, and Director and Chief Scientist, Complex Adaptive Systems Initiative, Arizona State University

WILLIAM ROUSE, Alexander Crombie Humphreys Chair and Director, Center for Complex Systems and Enterprises, Stevens Institute of Technology
WILLIAM STEAD, Chief Strategy Officer, Vanderbilt University Medical Center; McKesson Foundation Professor of Biomedical Informatics and Professor of Medicine, Vanderbilt University
CORNELIA ULRICH, Executive Director, Comprehensive Cancer Center, Huntsman Cancer Institute; Jon and Karen Huntsman Presidential Professor in Cancer Research, The University of Utah

NOTE: See Appendix C for Disclosure of Unavoidable Conflict of Interest.

Staff

GURU MADHAVAN (*Study Director*), Senior Program Officer, Health and Medicine Division (*through February 2019*); Director of Programs, National Academy of Engineering (*from February 2019*)
FRANCIS AMANKWAH, Associate Program Officer
ANNALEE GONZALES, Senior Program Assistant
SHARYL NASS, Director, Board on Health Care Services and National Cancer Policy Forum

Consultants

MICHELE McCORKLE, University of Pittsburgh
ROBERT POOL, Editorial Consultant
BRENDAN SALONER, Johns Hopkins Bloomberg School of Public Health

Reviewers

This Consensus Study Report was reviewed in draft form by individuals chosen for their diverse perspectives and technical expertise. The purpose of this independent review is to provide candid and critical comments that will assist the National Academies of Sciences, Engineering, and Medicine in making its published report as sound as possible and to ensure that the report meets institutional standards for objectivity, evidence, and responsiveness to the study charge. The review comments and draft manuscript remain confidential to protect the integrity of the deliberative process.

We thank the following individuals for their review of this report:

NORMAN R. AUGUSTINE, formerly Lockheed Martin Corporation
LOUIS P. GARRISON, University of Washington and formerly ISPOR
JEFFREY P. KOPLAN, Emory University
TRACY A. LIEU, Kaiser Permanente
HAMILTON MOSES III, Alerion Advisors, LLC; formerly Boston Consulting Group; and formerly Johns Hopkins Hospital
JOHN E. NIEDERHUBER, University of Virginia and Johns Hopkins University
NEELA PATEL, Seattle Genetics
ELIZABETH A. PLATZ, Johns Hopkins Bloomberg School of Public Health

HOLLY G. PRIGERSON, Weill Cornell Medicine
RINO RAPPUOLI, GSK Vaccines (Italy)
BARBARA K. RIMER, University of North Carolina Gillings School of Global Public Health
LEWIS G. SANDY, UnitedHealth Group
PATTI MIGLIORE SANTIAGO, Washington State Department of Health
JAY J. SCHNITZER, MITRE Corporation
LEE SCHWARTZBERG, West Cancer Center and University of Tennessee

Although the reviewers listed above have provided many constructive comments and suggestions, they were not asked to endorse the conclusions or recommendations, nor did they see the final draft of the report before its release. The review of this report was overseen by **DAVID R. CHALLONER,** University of Florida, and **ALFRED O. BERG,** University of Washington School of Medicine. They were responsible for making certain that an independent examination of this report was carried out in accordance with institutional procedures and that all review comments were carefully considered. Responsibility for the final content of this report rests entirely with the authoring committee and the National Academies.

Preface

Both my brother and my sister are cancer survivors, and I was my brother's bone marrow donor. Years of experience as a cancer surgeon and later as an administrator and chief executive officer of a hospital have given me extensive experience with cancer's medical toll, but this personal experience has shown me how the claws of cancer extend beyond the clinical setting, reaching into families, homes, and communities and taking far too much from far too many. Thus, it is doubly frustrating to me that our country—and, indeed, the world—has not made more progress against cancer than it should have.

Nearly half a century ago, the United States declared a "war on cancer" with the passage of the National Cancer Act of 1971. Even so, over the next 12 months in the United States alone, more than 1.7 million individuals will hear the devastating words, "You have cancer," and some 606,000 people will die from the disease—nearly twice as many as in 1971.

We have seen encouraging outcomes on several fronts, of course. For example, death rates from specific cancers have been steadily declining over the past 25 years, and fewer people are being diagnosed with certain cancers, such as lung and colorectal cancers. Still, with nearly 17 million cancer survivors in the United States today—and significant increases expected in the years to come—it is time to rethink our practice and systems of cancer control.

That rethinking needs to begin with a clear understanding of the status quo and the interests that prevail around it. The "system" of cancer control that currently exists in the United States has developed over time not under the direction of some master plan but rather piecemeal as the result of thousands of participants and their decisions. A clinician or hospital chose to get involved with cancer treatment. Oncology became a specialty of medicine, and further subspecialization occurred. Comprehensive cancer centers came into being. Federal agencies invested in research and introduced regulations. Companies developed many lifesaving products. Public health organizations started antismoking campaigns. State governments developed numerous cancer plans. Advocacy groups formed and worked for research funding, public awareness, or policy actions. Over time, the various entities and organizations developed various relationships among themselves. Today, cancer control in the United States is carried out by an extremely complicated, interconnected network of independent agents pursuing their own agendas and, when necessary or convenient, coordinating with some of the other agents in the network but otherwise having no hierarchical command structure or central decision-making body. Cancer control is, to use the principal term and guiding concept of this report, a complex adaptive system.

As has been true for decades, scientific and medical research is generating a steady stream of tools and insights for our cancer control arsenal. But today we have the opportunity to do something transformative for cancer control: leverage converging technologies and capabilities for the cancer control system to be more responsive to policy choices and be much more efficient and accountable overall. This change in our vision and approach is a crucial necessity given the large and growing cancer burden in the United States—a burden that currently comes to about $600 billion annually in terms of medical and related expenditures, as well as lost productivity, and could well approach $1 trillion in the coming years, not including social and other difficult-to-quantify costs. Indeed, many previous analyses and reports, including those from many of the groups I have been privileged to be part of, have starkly yet commonly concluded either that we have a "crisis" or that the situation, in which patients struggle to find ways to pay for cancer control, is "unsustainable." A starting point challenge is also the fact that the participants involved in cancer control operate in a multipayer universe without a single accountable authority and with different standards for acceptable evidence. Progress is both much needed and desired.

This report, *Guiding Cancer Control: A Path to Transformation*, starts with the complexity of cancers and cancer control and then works toward motivating an approach that seeks to better understand, develop, and improve both our current and our planned efforts. This will require a robust integration of resources, efforts, and talents, an idea that is hardly novel—presidents from Franklin Delano Roosevelt to Richard Nixon and beyond have been committed to "conquering" cancer—but one that is still pressingly important. Cancers and cancer control efforts arouse financial and emotional energies across society, but going forward many of our strategies must necessarily be different.

Much of the work underlying this report began with a basic assessment of the following questions: Have we really made progress with cancer control? Are we asking and addressing the right questions? What needs to be done differently and better? How do we get all the people in the cancer control enterprise to communicate with one another, as well as collaborate?

At the outset of this study, these seemed like vague questions, but they sharply guided the vision for what "control" means or should mean. Historically, control has meant an emphasis on prevention, early diagnosis, and various treatments. This report begins with and builds on these but necessarily promulgates a wider conception of cancer control, starting from basic risk awareness through end of life, involving a range of participants broader than usually considered, and finally presents a national strategic vision for cancer control based on the scientific principles, engineering tools, and business and policy realities of complex adaptive systems. A novel contribution of this report, we believe, is in recognizing and documenting the variety of participants (especially within the U.S. federal government) focused on cancer control. This points to the continued need for integrated resources and activities across these agencies and other participants for which the report recommends the methods of systems engineering to achieve a greater degree of coordination in cancer control efforts.

Many committed and hard-working people involved in cancer control are responsible for the progress we have achieved. There are countless people alive today who owe a great debt to their efforts and the technologies they have developed and applied. Yet, ultimately, cancer prevails and continues to take a major toll on human life and suffering after 50 years of the "war on cancer." A driving reason could be that well-intentioned stakeholders in different fields have worked independently to make improvements in their specific areas of interest, but in today's world it is vitally essential—perhaps even a prerequisite—to understand and practice cancer control as a complex adaptive system and to develop strategies accordingly. In the future, decisions about cancer control ideally will be made after taking into account how changes will affect the entire system and not just one aspect of it, and this report offers specific suggestions for developing an approach to making such decisions.

The stakes now seem higher. The coming decades will see a sharp aging of the U.S. population and increases in costs associated with cancer control that could overwhelm the nation. The best bet for avoiding such a scenario is to approach cancers and cancer control as complex adaptive systems to transform our approaches, increase our accountability, and make best use of the talents and resources at our disposal. In doing so, not only can we improve the overall productivity of the nation and the lives of countless families—like mine—but also we can set a precedent to control other diseases.

—Michael M. E. Johns, *Chair*
Committee on a National Strategy for
Cancer Control in the United States

Contents

SUMMARY 1

1 COMPLEXITY: FROM CELLS TO SOCIETY 11
The Scope of Cancer Control, 12
Cancer Burden and Disparities, 15
Difficult Trade-Offs, 19
The Complexity of Cancers and Cancer Control, 22
The "Continuum" of Cancer Control, 24
Social Costs and Consequences, 33
Complex Adaptive Systems, 43
Findings, 50
References, 52

2 THE CURRENT "SYSTEM" OF CANCER CONTROL 63
Global Efforts in Cancer Control, 64
Federal Efforts in the United States, 67
State and Local Initiatives, 72
Performance Evaluation, 75
A Vigorous System of Participants and Interests, 77
Consumer and Other Technology Firms in Cancer Control, 79
Historically Common Themes, 84
Public Trust in Cancer Control, 87
Toward a Consolidated Vision, 89
Findings, 90
References, 93

3 GUIDING THE SYSTEM OF CANCER CONTROL 101
Systems Engineering in Society, 102
Systems Approaches in Cancer Control, 105
Systems Analyses and Systematic Trade-Offs, 110
Building a Multi-Level Model, 117
Guidance Systems for Cancer Control, 121
Findings, 124
References, 125

4 A PATH TO TRANSFORMATION 127
Conclusions, 128
Recommendations, 131
Applying the Guidance System, 135
From Many to One: Advancing the Practice, 137
Building New Capabilities and Competencies, 142
Working for Success, 143
Setting a Precedent, 145

APPENDIXES
A STAKEHOLDER INPUT 147
B BIOGRAPHICAL INFORMATION 149
C DISCLOSURE OF UNAVOIDABLE CONFLICT OF INTEREST 159

Summary

The challenge of cancer control starts with the complex nature of cancers themselves. Throughout history, few other diseases have generated the level of social, scientific, and political discourse or have had the degree of cultural significance as cancers. A collective in the truest sense of the word, "cancer" is a clustering of different diseases that afflict individuals in different ways. In the early 1970s, cancer was still largely thought of as a single target, albeit one that affected different parts of the body. Now, it is well known that cancer is a vast and evolving multitude of individual diseases with different biological mechanisms and different responses to treatments, but with a single overarching characteristic in common—the unchecked proliferation of the body's own cells. Cancers can occur in many human tissues and organs, and there may be many different subtypes that can be identified based on molecular abnormalities, yielding potentially hundreds of different types of cancers. Even what might seem to be a single cancer type—a cancerous lump in the breast, for example—can come in different versions that respond differently to a given treatment.

The burdens of cancers are also broad and diverse, from the physical, financial, and psychological tolls it imposes on individuals to the costs it inflicts on the nation's clinical care and public health systems. Decades of concerted efforts to understand and eliminate cancers, often referred to as the "war on cancer," have produced some significant advances in prevention (e.g., tobacco cessation and vaccines for hepatitis B and human papillomavirus), early detection (e.g., colonoscopy and cervical cancer screening), and treatment (e.g., targeted and combination therapies), but the burden of cancers is still substantial and growing as the population ages. Although age-adjusted cancer mortality has been steadily declining over the past three decades, about 600,000 people in the United States died from cancer in 2018, and about 1.7 million people received a new diagnosis of cancer. Moreover, significant disparities in cancer incidence and outcome persist across different populations.

The World Health Organization adopted a resolution in 2005 urging the member states to develop and reinforce comprehensive cancer control programs and evaluate their impact, and many countries now have a national cancer control plan. In the United States, however, cancer control efforts have evolved over time without a unifying national plan or centralized guidance. Numerous federal agencies have diverse roles in cancer control, but there is little cross-agency coordination, and each state and territory develops its own cancer control plan, with no overarching strategy or guiding vision of how an ideal cancer control system should operate or perform. Thus, the study sponsors (the American Cancer Society, the Centers for Disease Control and Prevention, and the National Cancer Institute) asked the National Academies of Sciences, Engineering, and Medicine to develop a national strategy for cancer control (see Box S-1). In response to that charge, a committee of independent experts appointed by the National Academies developed a set of recommendations that define the key principles, attributes, methods, and tools needed to achieve the goal of implementing an effective national cancer control plan. In developing these recommendations, the committee reviewed literature on the history and current status of cancer control efforts in the United States and globally. In addition, the committee held two public sessions with sponsors and various stakeholders. The public sessions featured presentations and discussions focused on two overarching questions: "What have we learned in the past decade?" and "What should we be doing differently?" These meetings provided an opportunity for the committee to seek input from a broad range of experts in cancer control in the United States.

THE SCOPE OF CANCER CONTROL

A remarkable number of analyses have already been conducted on the subject of cancer control (perhaps more than for any other disease), with several dozen reports and proceedings issued by the National Academies alone over the past several decades. A National Academies report declared in 2013 that cancer care in the United States was in "crisis." That statement is no less true today and can be generalized to the full spectrum of cancer control efforts. Hampered by poorly integrated resources, uncoordinated activities and conflicting interests and incentives, the current

BOX S-1
Statement of Task

An ad hoc committee under the auspices of the National Academies of Sciences, Engineering, and Medicine will examine cancer control efforts in the United States and recommend a national strategy to reduce the incidence, morbidity, and mortality from cancer and to improve quality of life for cancer survivors. The committee will review trends in cancer cases and outcomes in the United States as well as existing cancer control programs and initiatives across the cancer care continuum. Based on that review, the committee will consider potential actions to

- Establish comprehensive national goals for cancer control;
- Identify potential mechanisms to evaluate and advance progress toward these goals;
- Identify challenges to achieving these goals and highlight knowledge gaps that impede progress in cancer control;
- Foster collaboration and coordination among key stakeholders, clarifying roles in cancer control efforts, and to build on existing efforts and to develop and implement plans of action to overcome challenges; and
- Prioritize cancer control interventions that have the potential to achieve significant progress in improving population health and reducing health disparities.

The committee will issue a report with findings and recommendations to achieve progress in developing and implementing a national cancer control strategy.

cancer control system is underperforming in curbing the burden associated with cancers.

The causes and effects of cancers are complex, and addressing that complexity requires efforts across the continuum of cancer care, starting from basic risk awareness through the processes of cancer prevention, detection, diagnosis, and treatment, as well as palliative care, survivorship care, and hospice care, and all the supporting services linked to these efforts. Moreover, cancer control is affected in various ways by the environment, technologies, economics, policies, research quality, and ethics surrounding or transcending its more traditional aspects. These additional factors include such things as education, food quality and availability, and policies related to housing and urban development. Obviously, there will be no single solution that can succeed across a large percentage of cancers and populations. Therefore, the term "cancer control" as conceived and used throughout this report refers to a much broader range of actions than most people appreciate or practice; it comprises a variety of strategies and tactics aimed at helping people at risk for or diagnosed with cancers in various ways that can extend beyond the traditional notions of cancer prevention or treatment. This report also advances a strategic vision for transforming cancer control that would require a much broader alliance among federal agencies, state governments, and key participants in the for-profit, nonprofit, and other sectors, including the technology industry, with its growing investments in population health.

A SYSTEMS APPROACH TO ADDRESS THE COMPLEXITY OF CANCER CONTROL

The ability to systematically collect and analyze large volumes of data has advanced rapidly in recent years, and this has generated novel approaches to continuous, systematic learning and quality improvement in health care. For example, the learning health care system model strives to enable evidence-informed transformations by continually collecting and using data to systematically integrate new knowledge into care delivery processes and to improve outcomes and motivate greater collaboration among all participants. Other systems frameworks have also been used to assess and improve certain aspects of cancer control efforts across the continuum. A socioecological model, for example, has been used to examine the factors contributing to cancer disparities in communities with low-income residents. Although these models can be useful in understanding and improving certain aspects of cancer control, they are unable to holistically view cancer control efforts to obtain an overall perspective on the collective behavior of the numerous participants in the ecosystem.

To overcome the limitations of the current systems-based approaches to cancer control, the committee approached cancer control as a system of systems, with a focus on the concept of a "complex adaptive system." In short, a complex adaptive system is a system consisting of individual entities that act and interact with one another to advance their own "interests," modifying their behavior in response to what is happening in the rest of the system. The behavior of a complex adaptive system cannot be understood simply by examining its individual parts in isolation; instead, the overall behavior is a product of the way that the individual components influence one another. The hallmark of complex adaptive systems is that behaviors emerge that could not have been predicted by understanding the behaviors of the individual components. Examples of complex adaptive systems include not only ecosystems and living organisms but also national economies, transportation systems, and population health.

Tools from complexity science and systems engineering have been applied to systems such as manufacturing, banking, air traffic control, weather prediction, homeland security, and the Internet, to name a few. Like the cancer control system, most of these systems developed over time with no overarching "master plan" and with no one entity in charge, perhaps with many of the same practical challenges as in cancer control, such as how to integrate resources and capabilities and how to coordinate different components that are generally pursuing their own goals and interests. In the United States, multiple federal agencies are involved in cancer control in addition to those principally focused on health promotion, disease control, and medical benefits.

Systems engineering tools make it possible to analyze, understand, and predict the behavior of complex systems through the study of a system's components and how the interactions of those components produce the system's behavior. A detailed analysis is generally the first step in understanding a complex system, and it often involves creating models and simulations followed by rigorous testing to see whether the system's behavior under different situations can be reproduced. Once such a simulation has been constructed and tested, it can be used to test how the system will respond to various stimuli and changes, which in turn makes it possible to learn how to guide—not "command and control"—the system to a certain degree.

Although a search of the literature has uncovered no suggestions for using systems engineering approaches to understand the total system of cancer control, as this report is proposing, there have been a number of ideas and initial efforts related to the use of systems engineering concepts to understand individual components of cancer control. Published papers have discussed applying systems engineering techniques to cancer drug delivery, cancer survivorship, clinical care and patient safety, and efforts to reduce disparities in cancer outcomes. These precedents could inform a broader systems engineering approach to integrate the various resources and efforts currently in use for the nation's cancer control system, as can be observed through the varied work of at least 13 different federal agencies and numerous other participants in the for-profit and nonprofit sectors.

GUIDING THE TRANSFORMATION OF CANCER CONTROL

This report offers **10 conclusions** supported by **25 findings,** all based on the overarching message that overcoming the current narrow and uncoordinated approaches that significantly constrain progress and effectiveness across the segments of the cancer control continuum is an imperative. One of those conclusions emphasizes that cancer control needs to be **"recognized and approached in practice as a complex adaptive system whose elements are interactive and influential at multiple levels of society, starting with the individual. This change in mind-set is**

essential to recognize, reduce, and mitigate risks and make significant progress in diminishing the cancer burden in the United States, a situation challenged by aging and other demographic factors with no apparent blunting of costs across cancer control activities." The estimates of how much cancer control efforts cost vary, and it becomes a particularly daunting task to arrive at aggregate costs if one considers the complex adaptive nature of the disease and the efforts to control it. However, the total volume of expenditures attributable to, or associated with, cancer in the United States is estimated to be nearly $600 billion annually, and that figure will only increase with escalating cancer incidence due to an aging society and other factors, including behavioral factors. Therefore, a renewed vision to guide the development of new and more effective national approaches to cancer control is essential.

No single volume can issue detailed analyses and be comprehensive on every aspect of cancer control, and this report is no different. Indeed, this report has a different vision and ambition; it provides a higher level view on the progress made and yet to be made in cancer control and on what is still unclear about the various cancer control interventions and policy strategies. This report does not supply a construction blueprint that may be relevant only to one particular time, entity, or context because another conclusion of this report is: **"The design of a single top-down, static blueprint for cancer control programs and operations in the United States is currently neither realistic nor productive. Instead, greater effectiveness in cancer control requires centrally available customizable planning tools that are useful across contexts and that can actively support performance monitoring and accountability reviews. Dynamic data feeds, computational and other capabilities, and interactive visual analytics will be required for the supporting systems analyses."**

The necessity of this broader view is captured in another conclusion: **"The current processes and systems of cancer control are at best reactive to circumstances. A proactive and progressive planning system for cancer control policies and operations would necessitate a learning mind-set, from individuals to institutions, focused on periodically determining what activities should be initiated, expanded, or terminated, as well as critically analyzing the trade-offs and tracking the consequences of related decisions."**

The operational strategy recommended in this report will invariably require trade-offs, continuous learning, and adaptation as well as a diligent, accountable, and periodic review of initiatives and strategies going forward. Such a discipline might well be a national imperative in order to progressively tackle the wide-ranging effects of cancers. This report argues that the best chance for transforming the U.S. cancer control system is to apply such a systems engineering approach, and it sketches out what might be involved in such an approach, providing **three interlinked recommendations.**

RECOMMENDATION A: A U.S. National Cancer Control Plan should principally ensure resource integration and operational coordination across the various components of the cancer control system and should actively do the following:

1. **Improve, where feasible, effective, and affordable, the availability of preventive, screening, diagnostic, and therapeutic interventions. Encourage timely palliative care, hospice care, survivorship services, and related social services according to the preferences and values of patients and their families.**
2. **Leverage the advances in and apply "multi-omic" diagnostics to improve therapies and better understand their scientific, clinical, and economic impacts, including their role in creating additional new prospects for cancer control and overall cost reduction.**
3. **Integrate the use of social, behavioral, and other information made possible by the convergence of communication, social media, cognitive, financial, and sensor technologies as well as electronic health records, cancer registries, and insurance claims to establish large-scale interoperable data sources.**
4. **Use cloud computing, machine learning, and artificial intelligence tools for continuous analytics, rapid reporting of trends and patterns, and improved forecasting and performance reviews. Evaluate emerging data-intensive technologies not only for their utility in advancing health and economic parameters but also regarding their ability to protect individual privacy and the security of data systems.**
5. **Apply the tools of complex systems analyses for assessing the "value" of cancer control interventions, establishing robust policy and incentive assessments to guide the development and commercialization of products and services, developing new financing and payment mechanisms that alleviate overall cost burden, and aiding individual patients and their families in making informed decisions about cancer care.**
6. **Minimize the waste and harm stemming from disparate clinical practices, interventions lacking evidence of effectiveness, and conflicting clinical practice guidelines.**
7. **Track and monitor financial links, incentives, and disincentives throughout the processes and systems of cancer control and rigorously require conflict-of-interest disclosures across cancer care, research, and patient advocacy activities.**

8. **Expand and support reproducibility strategies for developing reliable evidence in cancer control from biomedical, clinical, public health, and social science research.**
9. **Discourage direct-to-consumer marketing and advertising of clinical products and services from companies, medical centers, intermediary firms, and other organizations by terminating the tax deductibility of these business expenses. Furthermore, tighten and enforce rules to particularly curb promotional tactics and strategies that are likely to mislead patients about the benefits of products and care services not based on strong evidence.**
10. **Launch and expand public engagement, literacy, and outreach activities, starting with K–12 curriculums and through technology platforms, to broaden the understanding of cancer prevention as an integral component of a healthy life course.**

Historically, cancer control efforts in the United States have prominently involved the federal government—featuring directions from the U.S. Congress or the executive branch—in launching new or expanded national initiatives. **Coordinating a wide range of federal agencies active in cancer control efforts could require congressional action if the participating agencies lack a legislative authority, in which case it is urged that the U.S. Congress provide the direction to implement the following recommendations.**

RECOMMENDATION B: A U.S. National Cancer Control Plan should be led by the Department of Health and Human Services in cooperation with the Office of Management and Budget, Department of Education, Environmental Protection Agency, Department of Defense, Department of Veterans Affairs, Department of Housing and Urban Development, Department of Agriculture, Social Security Administration, Department of Labor, Department of Commerce, Office of Personnel Management, Equal Employment Opportunity Commission, and Department of the Treasury. The Government Accountability Office should periodically review and report to the relevant congressional committees about the achievement of goals specified in the plan.

A national cancer control plan will need to include all these federal participants, as well as ongoing participation from state and local governments and key participants in the for-profit and nonprofit sectors to undertake a comprehensive review of diverse and shifting needs and an integration of available resources and capabilities. Periodic performance review and annual reporting, with a rigorous comprehensive review every 3–4 years, similar to the congressionally mandated assessments in other areas, would be essential for both improved accounting and accountability in cancer control. While this extensive level of cooperation may seem daunting, there is precedent for such an approach. For example, the U.S. Global Change Research Program, the NextGen air control system, biodefense initiatives, and intelligence community operations all require resource integration, joint monitoring, and diligent performance review across many different agencies, particularly involving industrial partnership. And, indeed, the iconic Apollo "moon shot" that has since inspired many activities of cancer control was a successful demonstration of more than 20 different government agencies cooperating under a congressional mandate. The ultimate success or failure of a national cancer control plan will depend on gaining a functional understanding of the nation's cancer control system and being able to predict how it responds to various interests and pressures. Therefore,

RECOMMENDATION C: To support a U.S. National Cancer Control Plan, the Department of Health and Human Services and the federal partner agencies should fund and support an independent organization—or a consortium—with principal competencies in systems engineering, industrial design, software development, and information and visual analytics to prototype and develop a publicly available, interactive, and evolvable planning and monitoring tool.

Moreover,
C-1: Periodic consultations with key participants from state and local governments, and for-profit and nonprofit sectors should focus on ensuring that data feeds to the planning tool are customized and routinely refreshed and that planning parameters are properly applied and extensively tested for transparency and meaningfulness.
C-2: Leaders from multiple sectors—biomedical, consumer products and services, computing, information technology, financial, transportation, agricultural, and construction—should be engaged through an advisory council mechanism.

It would be counterproductive and economically unfeasible if the various stakeholders each went about developing its own platform; hence the need for a "master version." The tool will also require as much up-to-date data about the nation's cancer control system as possible, so it will be important, for instance, that each state and territory use its own data—and refresh those data periodically for analyses and comparisons.

Large-scale tools such as this one envisioned for cancer control can be seen in regular use elsewhere in applications for monitoring, for example, the economy, weather, financial markets, labor dynamics, classified intelligence, and the manufacturing supply chain. Cancer affects everyone in one way or another. Thus, everyone has a stake in decisions about cancer control, which makes it crucial that the process of making those decisions be open and accountable. Successful national cancer control efforts will require a significant integration of resources and a major collaborative initiative among multiple participants to develop a joint ability with joint accounting and accountability. Using the science and engineering of complex adaptive systems offers productive possibilities for new progress in guiding the cancer control system to reduce the burden of cancers for individuals, families, and society as whole.

1

Complexity: From Cells to Society

For millennia, humanity has grappled with cancer, seeking both to understand it and to control it. The first documented mention of cancer was 3,500 years ago, when an Egyptian surgeon described treatmentts, usually unsuccessful, for breast cancer. Eleven hundred years later, the Greek physician Hippocrates thought that tumors of the breast resembled crabs and referred to them as *karkinos*, the Greek word for crab. Later, the Romans translated the term into Latin and called the tumors "cancer," the term we still use today. From the 15th through the 19th centuries, clinicians suggested a variety of causal explanations for cancers at different points of understanding, from "divine punishment," to noxious substances that spread through the body, or the product of lymph fluids (Sudhakar, 2009).

In the past century, cancers have become a very prominent threat to population health, in large part because people live long enough to have a higher likelihood of developing some type of cancer. During that same 100 years, the tools available to prevent, diagnose, and treat cancer have also multiplied. Eighty years ago, the only available treatments for cancer were surgery and radiation, but today's clinicians have many more options to treat their patients. Research over the past several decades has led to a much better understanding of the biology of cancer, albeit still incomplete, which in turn has led to rapid advances in prevention, detection, and treatments. Although benefiting many patients, these new technologies unfortunately have not mitigated the still substantial toll of cancer or led to the expected victory in the "war on cancer." In 2018, about 600,000 people in the United States died from cancer, and about 1.7

million people received a new diagnosis of cancer (Gapstur et al., 2018). According to the National Cancer Institute's (NCI's) "cancer clock," a new cancer is diagnosed in the United States approximately once every 30 seconds (NCI, 2018b).

THE SCOPE OF CANCER CONTROL

The goal of this report (see Box 1-1 for the study context) is to provide a national strategic vision for cancer control in the United States. In doing so, this report approaches "cancer control" as a much broader range of actions than is most commonly understood. The reason lies in the complex nature of cancer, which requires efforts on multiple fronts. Indeed, the history of cancer control can be seen as a gradual broadening of efforts, with the realization that each successive effort has not yet been sufficient to address the full spectrum of the cancer burden.

BOX 1-1
Study Background

The National Academies of Sciences, Engineering, and Medicine have a long track record (since at least 1928) in exploring strategies for cancer control. The National Academies have also conducted extensive analyses in advising the development of national (and at times global) strategic plans on various topics of science, engineering, and medicine, from aerospace technologies and maritime security to manufacturing and climate modeling. In health and medicine, National Academies publications have offered recommendations for national strategies to address HIV/AIDS and hepatitis and to prioritize health technologies such as vaccines.

To develop a national strategic vision for cancer control, the National Academies appointed an ad hoc committee of individuals[a] with a range of expertise and experiences, including epidemiology, clinical oncology, palliative care, cancer outcomes and survivorship, economics, ethics, evolutionary biology, engineering, and executive administration. The committee met twice in person, for 3 days each, in addition to convening online over numerous phone and video conferences. Two public sessions were held for stakeholder input as part of the study; the first one was a teleconference discussion with the study sponsors,[b] and the second one was a daylong public workshop.[c] The committee's Statement of Task can be found in the Summary in Box S-1.

---

[a] Appendix B contains biographical information, and Appendix C contains a disclosure of unavoidable conflict of interest statement.

[b] The study sponsors were the American Cancer Society, the Centers for Disease Control and Prevention, and the National Cancer Institute of the National Institutes of Health.

[c] Stakeholders who provided input are listed in Appendix A.

The earliest approach to treating cancer was exceptionally direct: excising it. One hundred years ago, this was the only option, and surgery to remove cancerous tissue did have some successes. But, in many cases, the cancer returned, often in a more aggressive version than the first time around. So in the mid-20th century, clinicians began working with radiation and drugs, generally in combination with surgery, to rid the body of the cancer. This was more successful, and clinicians gradually assembled an array of cytotoxic and molecularly targeted cancer drugs from which to choose for particular cases. More recently, clinicians have been working with immunotherapy, using the body's immune system to attack cancer cells. These various approaches—surgery, radiotherapy, chemotherapy, targeted therapy, and immunotherapy—constitute the "treatment" aspect of cancer control.

The realization in the 20th century that many cancer cases are not random occurrences but rather are the body's response to a particular carcinogen led to a second aspect of cancer control: "prevention." Such strategies as decreasing smoking rates and alcohol use, improving healthy food consumption, eliminating environmental carcinogens such as asbestos, and vaccinating against cancer-causing viruses such as the human papillomavirus (HPV) seek to prevent cancer from occurring in the first place.

If cancer does strike, the sooner it is detected, the better the odds are that a patient can be cured or effectively treated for some time. Thus, early detection is another important component of cancer control. Similarly, once a patient has—or is suspected to have—cancer, it is crucial to get an accurate diagnosis, as this points the way to the most appropriate treatment. The diagnostic aspect of cancer control involves physical examinations, imaging, laboratory tests on blood and other body fluids and tissues, pathological examinations of tumor tissues, and the analysis of this information to determine the likely stage and characteristics of the cancer.

Both the cancer itself and the treatment for it expose the patients and their families to all sorts of stresses—physical, financial, psychological, social, spiritual, and so on. Helping patients and their families deal with these stresses is not only the humane thing to do, but it may also influence the effectiveness of the treatment. Thus, the provision of such care has become accepted as another aspect of cancer control. Supportive services can help patients and their family members deal with a variety of psychosocial stresses, such as the depression that may accompany a cancer diagnosis or an extended course of treatment. "Palliative care" is focused on addressing the symptoms of cancer and the side effects of treatment, such as pain and nausea. It can, for instance, include the prescription of nausea-relieving drugs to help a patient deal with the side effects of chemotherapy or the use of radiation to shrink tumors that are causing pain or other symptoms, such as an incurable lung cancer triggering shortness of breath. As medical advances have allowed individuals with cancer to survive for increasingly longer periods, such palliative care has become a major aspect of cancer control. "Hospice care" refers to supportive and palliative care provided at the end of life. It is sometimes broken out as a separate aspect of cancer control. In recent years, as more patients are surviving a cancer diagnosis for long periods of time, many efforts have also focused on "survivorship care" to address the long-term and delayed effects from cancers and cancer treatment.

From Cures to Control

Formal policy approaches to reducing the cancer burden in the United States can be tracked back to 1928, when the U.S. Congress requested the National Academy of Sciences to provide advice to the federal government for developing "a successful and practical cure for cancer."[1] Nine years later, during the presidency of Franklin Delano Roosevelt, NCI was established by the U.S. Congress primarily to show "the useful application of results" (NCI, 2018c). NCI was scaled back during World War II, but in the postwar era, renewed interest in the subject led to the expansion of cancer control efforts (Breslow, 1979).

In 1971 President Richard Nixon signed the National Cancer Act, signaling the beginning of what was termed the "war on cancer." The act widely increased research on the biological basis of cancer, with the expectation of finding a cure. In addition to increasing federal expenditures on cancer research, the act significantly boosted the political and public profile of cancer. Since then, for instance, cancer surveillance capabilities have dramatically improved thanks to efforts of entities such as the National Program of Cancer Registries (which provides population-based cancer data for national, state, and local health planning),[2] and the federal Surveillance, Epidemiology, and End Results program (which established a coordinated system of cancer registries), complemented by efforts of private companies in the technology sector (White et al., 2017). As shown in Figure 1-1, the generally upward trend in cancer death rates evident through the early 1970s did not initially abate once the federal government had declared "war on cancer." Rather, mortality rates generally continued to increase for two decades before finally peaking around 1990. Since then, declines in age-adjusted mortality rates have been seen for specific high-incidence cancers: lung, colorectal, breast, and prostate. However, the statistics related to many other conditions, including

[1] S. 3554, 70th Congress, Sess. 1 (1928).
[2] This text has been revised since prepublication release.

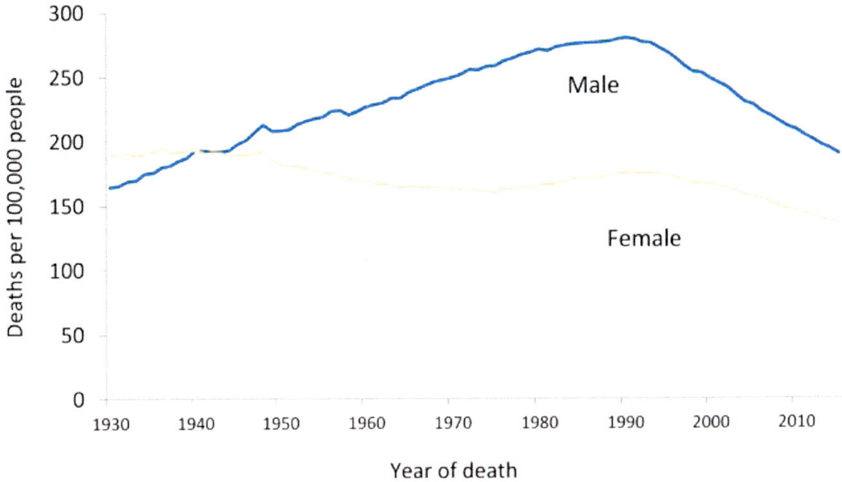

FIGURE 1-1 Trends in age-standardized cancer death rates among males and females in the United States, 1930–2015. Rates are age adjusted to the 2000 U.S. standard population and are presented per 100,000 person years. Data source: National Center for Health Statistics.
SOURCE: Siegel et al., 2018.

pancreatic, glioblastoma, and advanced metastatic cancers, have remained largely unchanged over time.

Generally speaking, the therapeutic approach to cancer has evolved from a purely "cures"[3] mind-set to a broader concept of "control." Although the general public, politicians, and many philanthropies still interpret the ultimate goal of cancer research as finding a "cure"—as indicated by the popular use of terms such as "conquests" or "moon shots" (inspired by the Apollo program)—in recent years, as noted earlier, various communities have begun to appreciate the need to find new avenues to better manage cancer as a chronic disease rather than focusing solely on elimination.

CANCER BURDEN AND DISPARITIES

Cancer control efforts face a vexing challenge due to the rapidly growing numbers of older people in the United States. As shown in

[3] The term "cure" is typically used to describe an outcome of a treatment where there are no traces of the cancer and where the cancer will never come back. Clinically, the term has been used to refer to conditions for persons whose signs and symptoms of cancer are reduced for 5 years or more. This concept, of course, is difficult to apply to all cancers because even after treatment, some cancer cells may still remain in the body and can cause complications later.

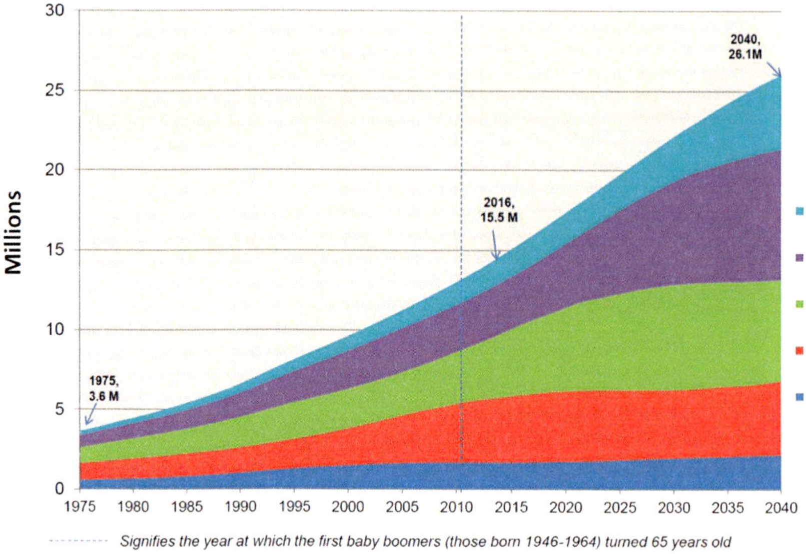

FIGURE 1-2 Estimated cancer prevalence by age in the U.S. population from 1975 to 2040.
SOURCE: Bluethmann et al., 2016. Reprinted with permission.

Figure 1-2, by 2040 the number of people in the United States aged 50–64 years with cancer is expected to be four times the number in 1975. The projected growth in the number of cancer cases is even more dramatic in older groups: a 6-fold increase in the 65–74 age range, a 10-fold increase for 75–84, and a 17-fold increase in the over-85 cohort (Bluethmann et al., 2016). The situation is due to the rapidly increasing numbers of people in older age brackets and not to increases in cancer rates among them. Concomitant increases in obesity rates are also expected to contribute to increased cancer diagnoses.

The burden of cancer can be observed most directly at the individual level. That burden is physical, emotional, psychological, social, and financial, and all these aspects are important, but it is the financial burden that can be most easily calculated. Cancer care, which is most often provided in outpatient settings,[4] comprises one of the largest cost components of clinical services in the United States (KFF, 2017), and expenditures on biopharmaceuticals and various care services have been growing. The financial burden of cancer care falls on a relatively small part of the

[4] See Table 3: Total expenses and percent distribution for selected conditions by type of service: United States, 2014. Agency for Healthcare Research and Quality. From https://bit.ly/2NsfCyd (accessed February 15, 2019).

population, with about 72 percent of cancer expenditures attributable to 5 percent of those with cancer (Cohen, 2014). Overall, 33 percent of cancer care expenditures during treatment are borne by Medicare and Medicaid, 44 percent by private insurance, and 15 percent through other sources (e.g., veterans' benefits), while only 4 percent of the cost of cancer care is actually paid (mainly through cost sharing) by the patients (ACS CAN, 2017). Still, that seemingly small portion can be a major burden. Nonreimbursed cost sharing for cancer care often leaves patients and their families with considerable debt as the percentage of cancer care costs fully paid for by insurance has been shrinking, and some patients may lack insurance altogether. One-third of patients undergoing cancer treatment go into debt (Banegas et al., 2016), and the costs associated with cancer care are one of the top reasons for declaring personal bankruptcy in the United States (Gilligan et al., 2018; Gordon et al., 2017; Lathan et al., 2016). Generally speaking, the economic impact of a cancer diagnosis will vary according to the features of the patient's insurance plan as well as the patient's ability to pay; furthermore, differences in patients' ability to pay is a major contributor to the disparities in cancer outcomes (ASCO, 2017; Gordon et al., 2017).

The incidence of cancer among minorities is also expected to grow much faster than among whites, with the latter expected to see the highest absolute number of cancer cases (because of their larger numbers in the population) but likely to have the smallest change in incidence—about 31 percent—over the 2010–2030 period. By comparison, cancer incidence is projected to increase by 142 percent for Hispanics, 64 percent for blacks, 132 percent for Asians/Pacific Islanders, 76 percent for American Indians/Alaskan Natives, and 101 percent for multiple-race individuals (Smith et al., 2009).

Cancer control efforts also exhibit persistent disparities in mortality rates among patients of different racial and ethnic groups, socioeconomic status, and geographic location of residence (Siegel et al., 2018) (see Figure 1-3). While the black–white differences in death rates during 1975–1980 for breast cancer and colon cancer (for both males and females) were relatively small, by 1990 (or before) the mortality rates for blacks far exceeded those for whites, and significant gaps remained through 2015. For prostate cancer, the mortality rate has declined consistently over the past 20 years, but it remains significantly higher for black men than for all other racial and ethnic groups.

Educational attainment is also known to affect cancer outcomes. In 2014 the risk of death for adults (aged 25–74) who had no more than a high school education was much higher than for those with at least a college education (for all major types of cancers except brain and other central nervous system tumors). There are also notable differences at the

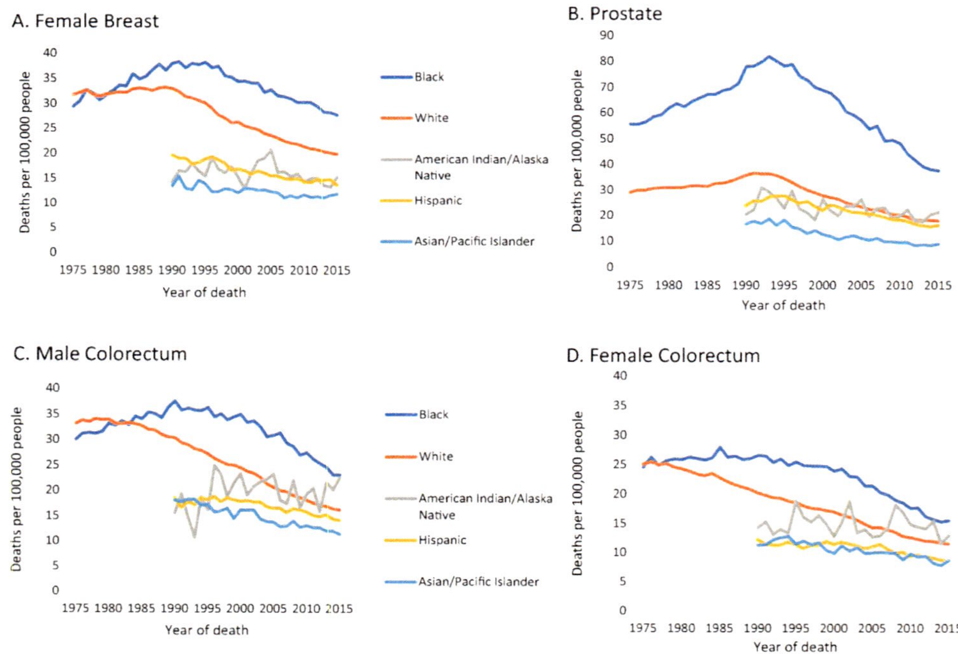

FIGURE 1-3 Cancer mortality by race/ethnicity from 1975 to 2015. Death rates are illustrated for (A) breast cancer (female), (B) prostate cancer, (C) colorectal cancer (male), and (D) colorectal cancer (female). Rates are per 100,000 and age adjusted to the 2000 U.S. standard population. Rates for American Indians/Alaska Natives (AIs/ANs) are based on the Contract Health Service Delivery Area counties. Rates for Hispanics exclude Louisiana, New Hampshire, and Oklahoma. Rates for whites, blacks, Asians/Pacific Islanders, and AIs/ANs are not exclusive of Hispanic origin. Data source: National Center for Health Statistics.
SOURCE: Siegel et al., 2018.

state and local levels in mortality rates for certain cancers, such as breast, colorectal, and lung. A classic example is the established link between smoking and lung cancer mortality rates at the state level, as shown in Figure 1-4. There are also important differences between men and women in the types of cancer they are likely to die from, as shown in Figure 1-5.

DIFFICULT TRADE-OFFS

The economic and clinical dimensions of cancer control present difficult resource allocation debates. One obvious issue is how to allocate health care

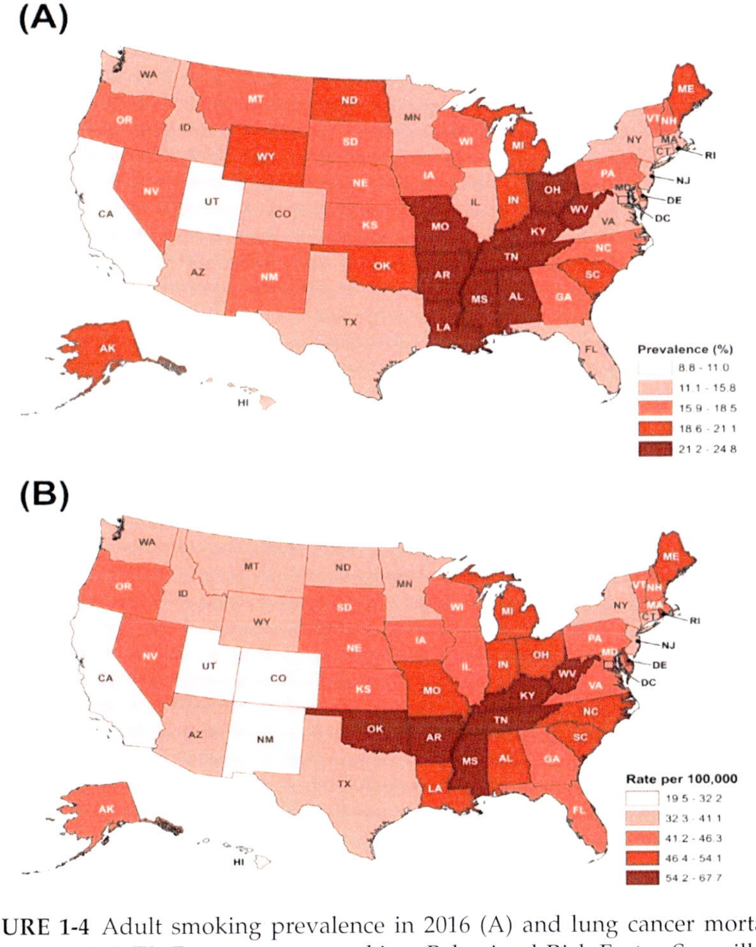

FIGURE 1-4 Adult smoking prevalence in 2016 (A) and lung cancer mortality rates 2011–2015 (B). Data sources: smoking: Behavioral Risk Factor Surveillance System, Centers for Disease Control and Prevention; mortality: National Center for Health Statistics.
SOURCE: Siegel et al., 2018.

Estimated New Cases

Male			Female		
Prostate	174,650	20%	Breast	268,600	30%
Lung & bronchus	116,440	13%	Lung & bronchus	111,710	13%
Colon & rectum	78,500	9%	Colon & rectum	67,100	7%
Urinary bladder	61,700	7%	Uterine corpus	61,880	7%
Melanoma of the skin	57,220	7%	Melanoma of the skin	39,260	5%
Kidney & renal pelvis	44,120	5%	Thyroid	37,810	4%
Non-Hodgkin lymphoma	41,090	5%	Non-Hodgkin lymphoma	33,110	4%
Oral cavity & pharynx	38,140	4%	Kidney & renal pelvis	29,700	3%
Leukemia	35,920	4%	Pancreas	26,830	3%
Pancreas	29,940	3%	Leukemia	25,860	3%
All sites	**870,970**		**All sites**	**891,480**	

Estimated Deaths

Male			Female		
Lung & bronchus	76,650	24%	Lung & bronchus	66,020	23%
Prostate	31,620	10%	Breast	41,760	15%
Colon & rectum	27,640	9%	Colon & rectum	23,380	8%
Pancreas	23,800	7%	Pancreas	21,950	8%
Liver & intrahepatic bile duct	21,600	7%	Ovary	13,980	5%
Leukemia	13,150	4%	Uterine corpus	12,160	4%
Esophagus	13,020	4%	Liver & intrahepatic bile duct	10,180	4%
Urinary bladder	12,870	4%	Leukemia	9,690	3%
Non-Hodgkin lymphoma	11,510	4%	Non-Hodgkin lymphoma	8,460	3%
Brain & other nervous system	9,910	3%	Brain & other nervous system	7,850	3%
All sites	**321,670**		**All sites**	**285,210**	

Estimates are rounded to the nearest 10, and cases exclude basal cell and squamous cell skin cancers and in situ carcinoma except urinary bladder. Estimates do not include Puerto Rico or other US territories. Ranking is based on modeled projections and may differ from the most recent observed data.

FIGURE 1-5 Ten leading sites of new cancer cases and deaths—2019 estimates.
SOURCE: Siegel et al., 2019.

spending among cancer and other conditions such as neurodegenerative and cardiovascular conditions, diabetes, opioid addiction, or acute epidemics. These needs, in turn, have to be evaluated against broader public service priorities such as the military, environmental protection, prison system, state and national parks, water supply, transportation systems, and other diverse forms of services. Between 2000 and 2014, the proportion of state budgets spent on Medicaid increased from 19 to 26 percent, forcing decreases in the proportions spent on other public programs (Joffe, 2015).

The "iron triangle" refers to access, quality, and cost containment in health and medicine (Kissick, 1994). Improvements are possible in one or two of these areas, but they will usually be at the expense of the third (Kissick, 1994; Lehman, 2015). The same observation applies to cancer control or to any of its individual components, from awareness of risks to providing hospice care for patients and bereavement support for families. This implies that there are inevitably trade-offs to be made when making decisions about cancer control investments.

For example, the median annual cost of a new cancer drug launched in 2017 had grown to more than $150,000 (IQVIA, 2018), and spending on prescription drugs, especially novel classes of targeted therapeutics and immunotherapies, has been among the chief contributors to rising national health expenditures in recent years (Martin et al., 2016; NASEM, 2018a). Cost figures of these sorts inevitably lead to discussions about how to best allocate finite resources in cancer control. For instance, the individuals who may benefit years from now from resources devoted to cancer prevention will be different from the individuals facing the need now for treatment of a diagnosed malignancy, which will often involve multiple therapeutic regimens. The people who could potentially benefit from cancer prevention are not readily identified when the investment is made, whereas there are identified patients who can directly benefit from care today. Moreover, there has been reluctance in the United States to adopt any scheme for stratification of access to care based on objective analyses of economic and clinical performance that might impose potential limits on care, a subject of intense political and media debate.

Cancer patients may face their own trade-offs, often having to decide between cancer treatment costs and meeting their other obligations, including other medical care (in addition to cancer care), mortgage, food, and other family expenses. Despite the fact that 96 percent of newly diagnosed patients with cancer have health insurance (Soni et al., 2018), the cost sharing poses practical challenges for patients whose expensive treatments are not completely covered by their insurers (Bernard et al., 2011; Claxton et al., 2018). The "financial toxicity" and the resulting psychological stresses associated with the exorbitant costs of cancer care are now a clinically recognized phenomenon (IOM, 2008; Meeker et al., 2016).

One study also reported food insecurity rates among cancer patients in New York City that were five times the state average (Gany et al., 2014). Clinicians have been hitherto reluctant to discuss the cost of care with their patients, and in particular they may tend to avoid direct discussion of the likelihood of successful treatment outcome in patients with advanced cancer. None of these questions is straightforward to answer.

THE COMPLEXITY OF CANCERS AND CANCER CONTROL

Cancers arise in different organs and progress and evolve in different time frames and trajectories. They involve diverse patterns of underlying clonal diversification and metastatic risk and have significant variation in their responsiveness to different classes of anticancer drugs. The etiology, taxonomy, and progression of different cancers are highly complex. Understanding this complexity is the first step to being able to transform cancer control efforts to achieve more effective outcomes at a lower cost for both society and individuals.

Classifications

Cancers vary widely from patient to patient, differing in the types of tissue affected, their causes and underlying biological mechanisms, their prognosis, and the most effective type of treatment. More than 200 different types of cancers—encompassing a vast diversity of malignant conditions—have been identified in humans. Each of these types of cancer itself has several constituent subtypes, yielding potentially several hundred more different types of cancers (Song et al., 2015).

Cancers are typically classified by the anatomic tissues or organs where they arise. For example, colon cancer is the result of malignant cell proliferation in the colon. But this pattern of naming does, at times, result in one term referring to many different conditions. For instance, "skin cancer" can refer to basal cell carcinoma, the most common form, which is relatively slow growing; the localized, low-grade squamous cell cancer, for which long-term survival may be nearly 100 percent; the more deadly melanoma; or several other less common types. The medical profession has followed this tissue-specific pattern in the way it divides itself into different specialties for the treatment of cancer (e.g., gynecologic oncology, genitourinary oncology), and specializing in such a way has allowed clinicians to hone their technical skills relative to a specific organ system. "Cancer staging" has also been used to classify cancers based on the tumor size, involvement of lymph nodes, and whether the cancer has spread to distant areas of the body (Edge and Compton, 2010).

Advances in genomics profiling and other molecular methods (e.g., epigenetics, proteomics, transcriptomics—collectively referred to as "multi-omics") are enabling a new molecular taxonomy for cancer (Chen et al., 2015; Idikio, 2011; Song et al., 2015). This reclassification of cancers could help provide refined insights into the underlying molecular pathologies in different cancer subtypes, which in turn could help clinicians in selecting treatment regimens tailored to individual patients. Another way of looking at cancers is by age: some clinicians and clinics specialize in pediatric cancers, while others specialize in treating cancers in adolescents, young adults, adults, and the elderly. There are a variety of other types of possible classifications as well. Those interested in public health might consider classifying cancers according to their ability to be detected early by screening (if that early detection could potentially lead to reduced mortality) or based on their associations with infections (e.g., cancers related to HPV or to hepatitis B and C). Some have also suggested classifying cancers based on modifiable risk factors (such as smoking, alcohol use, diet, and tanning beds).

Each of these approaches to cancer classification has its strengths and weaknesses. None is sufficient, on its own, for addressing all the complexities inherent in cancer control. That will require a wider, more comprehensive understanding of cancers and their burdens in place of the prevailing reductionist approach of narrowly understanding aspects of specific cancers. The challenge for those interested in reducing the cancer burden is to recognize that every approach to grouping cancers has limits and to develop strategies that can incorporate novel and effective ways of classifying, understanding, preventing, diagnosing, and treating cancer in order to gain the most comprehensive view possible—a subject that is discussed in detail in the latter sections of this report.

Representative Risk Factors

Another factor contributing to the difficulty of reducing cancer burden is the wide variety of things that can increase the risk of different types of cancer. This complicates efforts to predict and prevent it, to treat it, and to survive it. In brief, behavioral factors such as tobacco use, alcohol use, and certain dietary choices known to increase the risk of cancer are things that individuals have a certain amount of control over (WCRF/AICR, 2018). In recent years, the role of viruses and other infectious agents in increasing risk for certain cancers has also been established (as in hepatitis B and hepatocellular carcinoma) or better understood, as has the role of vaccines in curbing particular forms of cancers. HPV increases the risk of several types of cancer, most notably cervical cancer in women and cancer of the mouth and throat in both sexes (IARC, 2007). Vaccines that protect against the most common versions of HPV are available, but vaccination rates are lower than anticipated, for a variety of reasons (Attia et al., 2018; Dorell et al., 2011; Holman et al., 2014; PCP, 2018). Genetic mutations are also known to play a role in predisposition to certain cancers. The role of BRCA gene mutations in breast cancer is well known, but there are many others that affect a small portion of the population (Kuchenbaecker et al., 2017).

Environmental factors continue to play an important role in cancer as well (Hiatt and Brody, 2018; Jagai et al., 2017). For example, a recent review concluded that 16 percent of cancer deaths worldwide—and 36 percent of lung cancer deaths—can be attributed to environmental factors (Pruss-Ustun et al., 2017). Although there is still some debate about the precise estimates (Israel, 2010; PCP, 2010), there is little doubt that environmental exposures play an important role in the development of some cancers. Environmental sources of carcinogen exposures include indoor and outdoor air pollution and radon gas in buildings (IOM, 1999, 2002). Similarly, occupational exposures to carcinogens in mining, construction, manufacturing, and refining industries include asbestos, benzene, cadmium, chromium, arsenic, formaldehyde, and polycyclic aromatic hydrocarbons (IOM, 2006a). Agricultural workers may be exposed to carcinogenic herbicides and pesticides (Damalas and Eleftherohorinos, 2011). Although federal regulations have led to the removal of many of the worst carcinogens from the environment and workplace, others still remain, particularly in manufacturing and agriculture (Reuben, 2010).

Risk factors can interact to increase or decrease the likelihood of developing cancer in various ways, complicating cancer control efforts. For example, environmental exposure to radon gas is much more likely to lead to lung cancer in people who smoke than in those who do not (Méndez et al., 2011). Cancer-causing pollutants are also often found at higher levels in areas of lower socioeconomic status. Research on epigenetics, the mechanism through which some of these exposures affect the expression of cancer-causing genes, has enhanced understanding of cancer risk factors as well.

THE "CONTINUUM" OF CANCER CONTROL

In an attempt to bring some logical structure to the many different components of cancer control, the concept of a "continuum," illustrated in Figure 1-6, was developed (IOM, 2013a; NCI, 2018a). The continuum consists of a half dozen steps in cancer control that typically follow one another in a linear fashion: prevention, screening, diagnosis, treatment, survivorship, and hospice care, with palliative and supportive care cutting across these steps (IOM, 2013a). Despite the ideal that these various

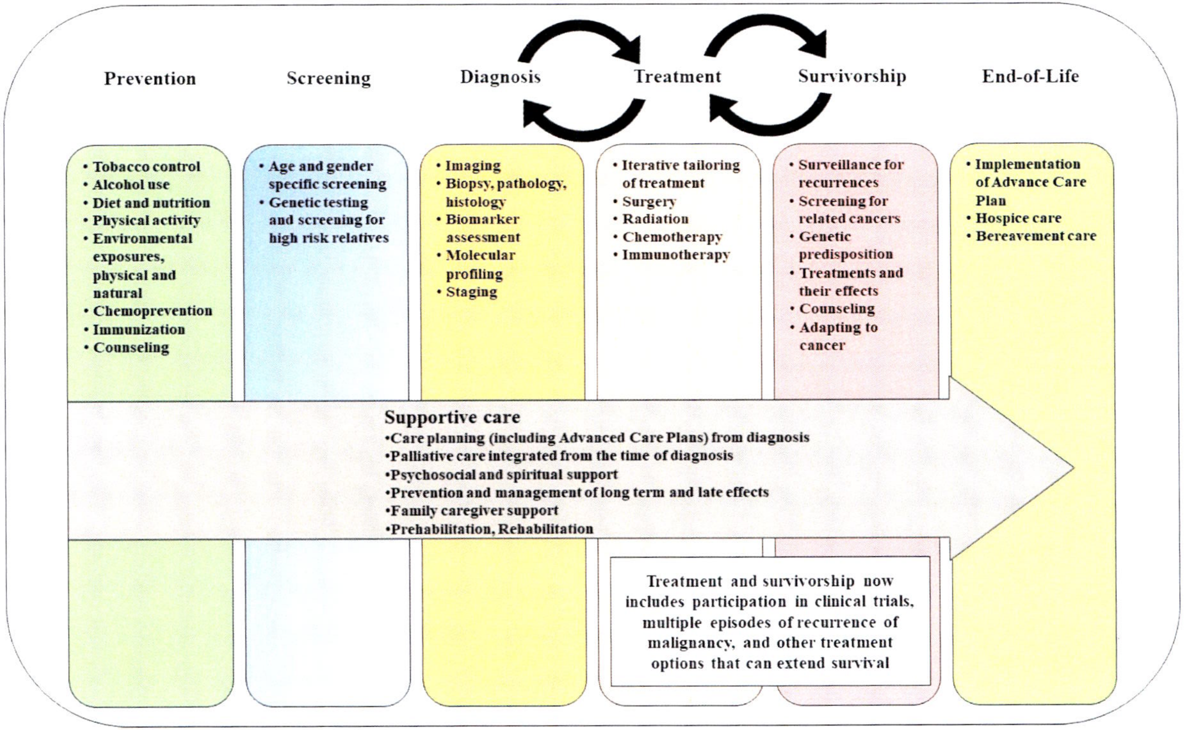

FIGURE 1-6 An individual-centric cancer control continuum reflecting a linear sequence of cancer control steps. Many external forces, including an aging population and financial constraints on individuals and society, have effects on this continuum.
SOURCES: Adapted from IOM, 2013a; NCI, 2018a.

steps should be connected, in practice it is often the case that specialists focus on the individual components separately, with little connectivity between them. As an example, survivorship is included in the continuum in recognition of the growing numbers of people alive with a history of cancer and of the specialized care needed to address the excess morbidity in these individuals. To emphasize the often episodic and recurring nature of treatment, the continuum now envisions a two-way relationship between treatment and survivorship (as people in the surviving population may transition back into treatment, and vice versa), similar to the coupling between diagnostics and treatments. Rehabilitation was once a specific phase, but it is now folded into treatment and survivorship care.

The components of "prevention" (the first block in the continuum) have expanded, starting with an increased awareness of various health-related behaviors that can be modified to reduce cancer risk and then with advances in chemoprevention, immunization, and prophylactic surgery, as in mastectomy in women at high risk for breast cancer (see Box 1-2).

BOX 1-2
Prevention and Risk Reduction in Cancer Control

The basic elements of cancer risk recognition, reduction, and mitigation have been classically pursued at three levels: primary prevention, secondary prevention, and tertiary prevention.

Primary prevention, which takes place before the onset of the disease, is aimed at preventing people from getting cancer in the first place, the most desirable outcome. According to estimates, about 42 percent of all cancer cases diagnosed in the United States and nearly half of all deaths from cancer are due to potentially avoidable factors, including tobacco use, unhealthy diet, alcohol intake, obesity, and physical inactivity (Islami et al., 2018). These risk factors have also been associated with other chronic diseases such as diabetes and cardiovascular diseases. Primary prevention methods include public awareness campaigns to encourage people to avoid behaviors that can increase the risk of cancers, immunizing against certain cancer-inducing viruses, removing carcinogens from the environment, and other health-promoting activities.

Secondary prevention involves the early detection and diagnosis of cancers so that they can be treated at a point when the treatment might be less harmful and has a greater chance of success. Tertiary prevention takes place after cancer has been diagnosed and is intended to reduce the complications and progression of cancer. Seen in this way, prevention is more than just a public health practice and directly extends into clinical care and rehabilitation.

The campaign to reduce smoking and the use of tobacco products has been arguably the most successful cancer prevention effort to date (CDC, 2018b; Singh et al., 2016). The multiple strategies have included product health warnings, media antismoking public service announcements, taxes on tobacco products, leg-

Components of "screening" (the second block in the continuum) now benefit from significant advances in genetic testing for high-risk relatives. Similar technological advances have also changed the profile of "diagnosis" (the third block in the continuum) to include improved imaging technologies and laboratory tests, including molecular profiling and biomarker identification. Surgery, radiation therapy, chemotherapy, targeted therapies, and immunotherapies have all played a significant role in advancing life-extending treatments[5] (the fourth block in the continuum; see

[5] A 2018 opinion survey from the American Society of Clinical Oncology noted that nearly 4 in 10 people in the United States believe that cancer can be "cured solely" through alternative therapies (ASCO, 2018). Additionally, users of alternative therapies say such therapies relieve them of side effects caused by their treatment and allow them to have control in their treatment (Bardia et al., 2006; Snyderman and Weil, 2002). Despite the growing use and awareness of these complementary and integrative health interventions—currently a $34 billion market in the United States (NCCIH, 2018)—very little analysis has been focused on the safety, standardization, regulatory, legal, and payment mechanisms for these approaches.

islative bans on tobacco advertising, and bans on smoking in college campuses and various public places (Glantz and Balbach, 2000). As a result, smoking rates among U.S. adults have declined steadily over the past decades. Nonetheless, 14 of every 100 U.S. adults still smoke (CDC, 2018a), and the recent decline in smoking has been accompanied by an increase in the use of alternative nicotine delivery products, such as e-cigarettes, for which the long-term effects remain unclear (Allen et al., 2018; Foulds, 2015; Liu et al., 2017; NASEM, 2018b). Cigarette smoking (including secondhand smoke) has been estimated to be responsible for approximately 20 percent of all malignancies and about 30 percent of all cancer-related deaths in the United States (Islami et al., 2018; Jacobs et al., 2015; Lortet-Tieulent et al., 2016).

In contrast with antismoking efforts, relatively little progress has been made in decreasing the cancer risks posed by diet, obesity, and alcohol consumption. Part of the reason is that the relationship between these other risk factors and cancer is not as straightforward as is the case with smoking, and the activities involve social customs and preferences as in the case of diet and alcohol (much like how smoking at one point was considered a refined social habit).

The World Cancer Research Fund has provided 10 lifestyle recommendations for preventing cancers (WCRF/AICR, 2018), with a key focus area being healthy weight management, because obesity is expected to overtake tobacco use as a lead risk factor for cancer (NASEM, 2017). Recent work (Booth et al., 2001; Owen et al., 2010; Sallis et al., 2006) has also sought to better understand behavioral influences at various levels beyond individual responsibilities, such as nutritional intake and sedentary lifestyle, to include the roles of social network influences and the availability of transportation options in a community. Some related policy concepts that have been proposed (and implemented in some areas) include insurance reimbursement programs that incentivize healthy lifestyle choices (Coughlin

continued

BOX 1-2 Continued

and Keckley, 2013; Lunze and Paasche-Orlow, 2013), expanding physical education and healthy food offerings in schools (Olstad et al., 2017), the taxation of sugar-sweetened beverages (Backholer and Martin, 2017; Hagenaars et al., 2017), federal dietary statements (Huang et al., 2018), and city planning initiatives that improve the walkability of U.S. cities (Berrigan et al., 2015).

A challenge that emerges from the numerous studies that have looked at the relationship between diet and cancer is that while it is clear that obesity is associated with an increased risk of certain types of cancers, these associations are not strong (Gonzalez and Riboli, 2006; Martinez et al., 2008; McCullough and Giovannucci, 2004). Thus, as difficult as it was to convince people to stop smoking—or to never start—in order to decrease their cancer risk, it is even harder to convince people to lose weight, drink less alcohol, or exercise more as a way of lowering their chances of cancer. (Reproducibility is a crucial condition for the generation of reliable scientific evidence. This topic is discussed further in Chapter 2.)

Secondary prevention includes cancer screening to diagnose cancer early. Early detection and diagnosis of certain cancers have been shown to improve cancer survival rates significantly and have been estimated to save up to $2 billion in treatment costs annually (Kakushadze et al., 2017). Many organizations

Box 1-3). In recent years, the ability to generate multi-omic information and the availability of advanced computational tools has fostered a growing emphasis on precision medicine approaches for cancer treatments.

Treatments are coupled with the next (fifth) block in the continuum, "survivorship,"[6] a topic that has garnered more appreciation in recent decades (Brown and de Graaf, 2013; Gibson et al., 2016). Survivorship also includes surveillance for recurrence and attention to acute and chronic effects of treatments, which can affect a patient's quality of life (see Box 1-4). This spectrum also captures a strong coupling between "treatment" and "survivorship." Cancer care has now progressed to the point that

[6] There is no uniform or universally accepted definition of who a cancer survivor is (IOM, 2006b). Attempts to define this term are commonly based on factors such as the stage of the disease, the progression of the disease across the different phases of the continuum, and the outcome of the disease after treatment (Marzorati et al., 2017). Furthermore, the heterogeneous nature of cancers—and the differing outcomes—makes it very complicated to understand when survivorship begins. Many consider survivorship as beginning at the time cancer is identified in the body and continuing through the remaining years of life. Others believe that survivorship stretches from cancer treatment until cancer recurrence or end of life. This term "survivor" was expanded in the national action plan for cancer survivorship to refer to "those people who have been diagnosed with cancer and the people in their lives who are affected by their diagnosis, including family members, friends, and caregivers" (NCI, 2019).

have published cancer screening and care guidelines, as discussed in Box 2-3. As new cancer screening approaches and tools emerge for the early detection of various cancers, it will be continually important to put in place quality standards for all screening tests, whether based on laboratory tests or imaging, in order to ensure that the potential benefits of early detection outweigh the potential harms for patients.

Cancer prevention efforts are being steadily improved because of research advances in molecular epidemiology, monitoring environmental exposures, and understanding the contributions of infectious diseases and lifestyle. But socio-cultural factors can frustrate even simple and effective prevention measures. A comparison of national receptiveness to vaccination against human papillomavirus (HPV) in the United States and Australia is instructive. In Australia, a national HPV vaccine program has achieved very high rates of coverage in the population, with the projection that cervical cancer could largely be eliminated as a public health problem there within the next two decades or so (Hall et al., 2018). The United States, by contrast, lacks a coordinated national effort for HPV vaccination and has faced political and religious opposition and litigation (for instance, with concerns that the vaccines will affect teen sexual behavior) (Abiola et al., 2013). A recent report from Canada, however, indicates that HPV vaccines there have served as effective tools to improve public health awareness among teens (Ogilvie et al., 2018).

many survivors live long enough to experience secondary or related cancers or a recurrence of their initial cancer. Cancer survivorship is often accompanied by long-term or delayed effects of treatment. The sixth block of the continuum is hospice care (IOM, 2015), which can be used for the greatest benefit if health care providers have a good system of timely referral of patients to hospice care, rather than days or weeks prior to death. Despite the desire of most patients to die at home, many often spend their final days in clinical settings. Early and ongoing conversations about end-of-life care between patients and their clinicians have shown to be beneficial for both patients and their families (Epstein et al., 2017; Wright et al., 2008).

The total cost of cancer care delivered in the last weeks or days of life is substantial (Wang et al., 2016; Zhang et al., 2009). Much of this care, however, may not be consistent with patients' wishes. Aggressive cancer treatment delivered in the last days of life has also been associated with poor quality of life and a worsened quality of death (Prigerson et al., 2015). Many recent analyses and efforts have focused on expanding the use of advance directives, enhanced spiritual and psychosocial counseling, and clinician education to improve communication with dying patients and their families (El-Jawahri et al., 2018; Riedel et al., 2017).

BOX 1-3
Advances in Cancer Therapies

Current cancer treatments rely on decades of advances in diagnostic imaging and pathology, surgery, multiagent chemotherapy regimens, molecularly targeted therapies, immunotherapy, and radiation therapy. Diagnostic imaging techniques have been steadily increasing anatomic resolution to locate increasingly smaller cancers and also include advanced abilities to monitor the metabolic or molecular signals of tumors. These capabilities have helped identify cancers at earlier stages and better characterize the local invasion or distant metastasis to design relevant treatment regimens.

The use of combination chemotherapy regimens has increased survival and cure rates for patients diagnosed with certain cancers. In the 1970s, for example, testicular cancer was fatal within 1 year of diagnosis for 95 percent of incident cases. With the introduction of cisplatin-containing chemotherapy regimens, 95 percent of patients with that disease are cured (Hanna and Einhorn, 2014; NIH, 2018).

Advances in radiation therapy, such as intensity-modulated radiation therapy, stereotactic radiotherapy, and proton therapy, have allowed highly precise and conformal delivery of radiation therapy to tumors while minimizing normal tissue exposure and its accompanying side effects (Jawerth, 2018). Immunotherapies now harness a patient's own immune system to effectively fight many types of cancer (Koury et al., 2018). Approaches are being developed to manipulate the human immune system to counter the complex adaptive capabilities of cancer cells by inhibiting immune checkpoints that prevent the body from attacking a cancer or through specific antibodies against cancer cells. Using the host's own immune system to fight cancer has now been taken a step further via development

The continuum also recognizes the fact that patients and families require extensive support, as indicated by the shaded arrow cutting across the blocks of the continuum. A major shift in cancer control has been the important focus now being placed on palliative care to address symptoms and side effects (including delayed effects) from the time of diagnosis, coupled with psychosocial and spiritual support. Palliative care is considered to be most effective when it is implemented early in the course of illness and its use is communicated and applied across all stages of diagnosis, treatment, survivorship, and disease recurrence (Ahluwalia et al., 2018; Ferrell et al., 2017; Gaertner et al., 2017). Recent guidelines have stated that the comprehensive assessment and management of symptoms is as important as attending to social, spiritual, and cultural considerations at the time of a person's death (Ahluwalia et al., 2018; El-Jawahri et al., 2018; NCHPC, 2018). The needs of family caregivers are also increasingly a subject of consideration (Lobb et al., 2015).

of adoptive cell therapy, whereby a patient's tumor along with critical cancer-fighting immune cells are harvested. These immune cells are manipulated and augmented, then reinfused into the patient to form a personalized antitumor immune response—an approach considered promising but resource intensive (Rosenberg and Restifo, 2015). Furthermore, tools for cancer diagnosis and treatment monitoring are being advanced toward the detection of microscopic evidence of cancer's presence or recurrence with a blood test. This "liquid biopsy" technology is currently under development to allow highly sensitive, rapid, simple, and relatively affordable cancer biomarker detection in the bloodstream (Liu et al., 2018).

The rationale for new and emerging technologies for cancer treatment is often described in literal "rocket science" terms, such as "moon shots," which is increasingly thought to be a misapplied metaphor for cancer. Instead, the effectiveness of any cancer treatment—or cancer control intervention—is wholly dependent on the complex system that adopts that intervention. Examples of variation in the application of cancer interventions by nonclinical factors have been found in analyses of data from the Surveillance, Epidemiology, and End Results–Medicare database. For example, one early study showed that whether a patient received recommended radiation therapy for breast cancer was associated with whether the patient was enrolled in a health maintenance organization versus fee-for-service insurance plan (Riley et al., 1999). Similar studies have shown that hospice enrollment and the quality of care at the end of life varies by race or type of insurance payer (Guadagnolo et al., 2014, 2015; Hardy et al., 2011). These are just a few examples of how the promise of treatments for certain forms of cancer control may also be blunted by unwarranted variation in clinical practice and reimbursement policies.

The continuum has been acknowledged as an oversimplification of both the biology of cancer and the clinical services needed (IOM, 2006b). The segmented phases shown in the continuum are not discrete. For example, a colonoscopy offers a valuable point of prevention via both the detection and the removal of precancerous polyps. Although external forces influence each component of the continuum (e.g., the role of neighborhood or even larger communities), their importance is rarely acknowledged in research and clinical practice (Stange et al., 2012).

Second, the continuum may not yet fully address the needs of cancer survivors. One report estimates that 80 percent of children diagnosed with cancer will now become long-term survivors (Campo et al., 2011), but these children have a substantially elevated risk of developing a second malignant neoplasm and other chronic health conditions (Bowers et al., 2013). Survivorship is thus not an end point (after which an individual is "cured" of cancer) but rather an ongoing process that may require lifestyle

BOX 1-4
Survivorship Support Services

The transition from cancer "patient" to cancer "survivor" has been a subject of recent focus (Miller et al., 2016). Of the estimated 16 million cancer survivors in the United States, a substantial number are likely to be at risk for morbidity, reduced quality of life, and premature death (IOM, 2006a; Miller et al., 2016). These long-term and late effects of treatments are known to affect physical (e.g., cardiovascular, second malignancies), psychosocial (e.g., fear of recurrence, depression), and practical (e.g., employment difficulties, financial issues) matters (Miller et al., 2016). Numerous organizations have called for specific attention to these concerns and care guidelines (Cohen et al., 2016; El-Shami et al., 2015; NCCN, 2018; Runowicz et al., 2016; Skolarus et al., 2014). Recommendations have included psychosocial support, educating the workforce, the evaluation of novel models of care, and addressing the financial burden of cancer care (Kline et al., 2018). Recently updated palliative care clinical practice guidelines have also emphasized four of the most important tenets of quality survivorship care: comprehensive assessment, effective pain and symptom management, good communication between patients and clinicians, and care coordination during transitions (NCHPC, 2018). For example, pain is frequently reported by cancer survivors as an uncontrolled symptom. In a study of head and neck cancer survivors, 45 percent reported pain, and of those individuals with pain, 46 percent reported a low quality of life (Cramer et al., 2018).

The majority of cancer survivors are over the age of 65 and do not receive medical care from a cancer specialist 5 years after their diagnosis (Pollack et al.,

changes, ongoing medical care, and treatment and support for reemerging complications as well as financial matters of care. The continuum can thus be criticized for engendering an unrealistic expectation of how individuals ultimately progress through cancer care; misperceptions of cancer care as a time-limited event rather than as an ongoing life experience can be detrimental in how cancer risk factors (and prevention) are communicated to the public and to the survivor community in particular.

Finally, each step in the cancer control continuum involves a wide range of participants, including patients; the patients' families, caregivers, and communities; clinicians; health systems; and insurers. The dilemma is that the contributions of these different constituencies are typically not well coordinated and may have widely varied incentives and conflicts of interests. The cancer control continuum, however, still provides a baseline to discuss the evolution of a national strategic vision for cancer control, with Table 1-1 providing a set of representative knowns and unknowns in practice.

2009). They transition their survivorship care to a nononcology primary care clinician. A study assessing the needs of long-term cancer survivors—which included 5- and 10-year cancer survivor cohorts—identified pain and sexual dysfunction as concerns in more than one-third of those survivors (Burg et al., 2015). Older cancer survivors preferred maintaining autonomy and independence while dealing with physical and functional limitations—one of the many points that suggest the need to improve survivorship care skills as a specific clinical competency (Guerard et al., 2016; Rubinstein et al., 2017; Thom et al., 2019).

The state of pediatric cancer survivorship care also requires specific clinical competencies. Survivors of childhood cancers are uniquely vulnerable to developing severe, life-threatening, treatment-associated conditions and late-onset complications resulting from cancer treatments. Pediatric cancer survivors also may have growth or developmental delays related to their treatment that can impede psychosocial function. Children may develop emotional attachment to their pediatric oncology team, which may not be the best source of health care to meet their needs as they transition to adulthood. However, one study assessing readiness of adult care facilities to care for pediatric cancer survivors reported that a lack of relevant competencies posed a serious barrier to transitioning childhood cancer survivors to adult primary care (Kenney et al., 2017). The need for more attention to improve the transition from "childhood cancer survivor" to an "adult survivor of childhood cancer" is a point of active discussion in the specialist communities, particularly regarding the unique physical and psychosocial needs of these patients (Frederick et al., 2017; IOM, 2003).

SOCIAL COSTS AND CONSEQUENCES

To appraise the costs and economic consequences of future cancer control efforts, it is important to understand the current magnitude of the aggregate cancer cost burden in the United States, including spending on cancer control. Addressing this daunting question is all the more challenging because of the complex nature of the disease, the multiplicity of cancer control activities under way, and the absence of organized efforts to identify, collect, and aggregate total spending from all agencies, organizations, and firms engaged in cancer control. The economic cost of cancer comes in many forms. There are the cancer-related health care costs across the cancer continuum (prevention, diagnosis, treatment, survivorship, and end of life); resources devoted to allied support services (including by the nonprofit sector); expenditures on research (both government and industry); and spending on wellness-promotion activities (by firms across the economy and by individuals seeking to stay cancer free). In addition, both the premature mortality and excess morbidity attributable to cancer impose significant productivity costs from a societal perspective (and, in

TABLE 1-1 Some Knowns and Some Unknowns Across the Practices of the Cancer Control Continuum

Interventions	Some Knowns	Some Unknowns
Prevention	– Risks imposed by tobacco use, obesity, and alcohol use (Connor, 2017; Griswold et al., 2018; Kerr et al., 2017; Mayne et al., 2016) – Cessation of tobacco use in reducing the risk of lung cancers (Cataldo et al., 2010; Clancy, 2014) – Effectiveness of hepatitis B and HPV vaccines in preventing liver and cervical cancers (Lowy and Schiller, 2012) – Effectiveness of certain oral drugs in reducing the risk of certain subtypes of breast and colon cancers (e.g., tamoxifen, aspirin) (Steward and Brown, 2013)	– Pathways of cancer risk factors such as obesity and alcohol use (LoConte et al., 2018), environmental carcinogens (Kiadaliri et al., 2013) – Measures to scale prevention strategies—from "precision" to population approaches – Measures to expand approaches to improve risk awareness – Economic characterization of preventive strategies on overall reduction of cancer burden – Reliable evidence concerning the role of diet and nutrition – Role of housing and taxes, among other policies
Screening, Detection, and Diagnostics	– Effectiveness of certain screening tests for most types of breast, colorectal, cervical, and lung cancers (Smith et al., 2018) – The risk of overdiagnoses and their adverse consequences (Brodersen and Siersma, 2013; Ong and Mandl, 2015; Welch et al., 2016) – Potential of genetic testing shown in certain kinds of hereditary cancer types (Rosenthal et al., 2017)	– Measures to improve uptake of effective screening, detection, and diagnostic strategies (O'Dowd and Baldwin, 2017) – Differentiating aggressive and nonaggressive tumors (Li, 2012) – Efficacy of molecular profiling and other advanced techniques – Cost control measures – Reproducible evidence for effectiveness of screening, detection, and diagnostics

TABLE 1-1 Continued

Interventions	Some Knowns	Some Unknowns
Treatment	– Cures of gestational trophoblastic disease and testicular cancer and early stages of certain types of breast and lung cancers – Increased survival outcomes for certain subtypes of lymphoma, lung and breast cancers (e.g., chemotherapy combination regimens) – Chemotherapy-sparing agents that specifically target oncogenic pathways (e.g., imatinib in chronic myeloid leukemia) – Effective radiotherapy to contour cancerous tissues while sparing normal tissues – Improved management of side effects (Spallarossa et al., 2018)	– Full benefits of therapeutic vaccines – Clinical trial end points for better assessment of survival – Prevention of secondary cancers as a consequence of treatment – Prevention of metastatic disease following initial treatment – Clinical and long-term value of precision medicine – Clinical effectiveness of prognostic and predictive biomarkers across cancer subtypes – Improving quality of life following treatment – Establishing guidelines for delivering less aggressive care – Strategies to mitigate cost burdens for patients diagnosed with cancer – Strategies to improve efficiency, reproducibility, and cost of cancer clinical trials
Survivorship	– Approaches to preserve functionality and reproductive potential following treatment – Measures to alleviate side effects	– Better management of long-term psychosocial effects of diagnoses and treatment – Role of diet and nutrition – How to improve communication with family members of inherited cancer risk – Full potential of cancer survivorship care plans (Jacobsen et al., 2018)
Palliative Care and End-of-Life Care	– Integrating palliative care in earlier disease stages (IOM, 2013a) – Respecting patient preferences and values – Effectiveness of advance care planning	– Improving approaches for communicating the benefits of palliative care – Establishing guidelines for delivering less aggressive care – Societal implications of individual care – Cost and resources involved in symptom alleviation throughout the care continuum

parallel, lead to lost or reduced incomes for individuals and families affected by cancer).

In what follows, a range of published data sources and modeling assumptions are used to arrive at a rough estimate of the total annual economic cost of cancer in the United States, from the broadest national perspective. The focus first is on cancer-related direct medical costs and indirect (productivity) costs. Then order-of-magnitude estimates are derived for additional public- and private-sector spending that may not be routinely reported (or even computed) but are clearly aimed at enhancing cancer control efforts.

First, regarding direct medical costs, NCI has projected that the net cost of cancer care for the United States in 2020 could be $173 billion (Mariotto et al., 2011) under specific assumptions about trends in cancer incidence, survival, annual increases in the cost of care, and changes in the size and age structure of the U.S. population over time. This projection includes expenditures associated with diagnosis, treatment, survivorship, and end of life—but not for screening/early detection nor for primary prevention, so in that sense can be regarded as a conservative projection of total cancer-related direct medical costs.[7]

---

[7] Based on data from another recent analysis of total medical care spending in the United States (Dieleman et al., 2016), one could derive (in several steps and under certain assumptions) an alternative projection of cancer-related direct medical costs for 2020 of about $147 billion. The study by Dieleman and colleagues and the analyses by NCI were both systematically executed though relying on a different mixture of data sources. NCI results are employed here, in part because they are directly derived 2020 cost projections, based on statistical modeling analyses that took into account projected changes over time (from 2010 through 2020) in cancer incidence, survival, the cost of care, and the size and age structure of the population.

While there are evidently no published estimates of the total annual cost of cancer screening/early detection in the United States, recent studies focused on individual cancer types may be informative. For example, one analysis using multiple data sources (principally the Behavioral Risk Factor Surveillance System Survey and Breast Cancer Surveillance Consortium data) and modeling assumptions estimated the annual total cost of breast cancer screening to be $7.8 billion (O'Donoghue et al., 2014). Another analysis by Gross and colleagues (2013) using different data sources (principally SEER-Medicare) estimated the annual costs of breast cancer screening-related procedures (screening plus workup) to be $1.08 billion (2009 dollars) for the fee-for-service Medicare population only. Considering that national-level estimates of the total cost of cancer screening should also encompass the other major screen-detectable cancers (colorectal, cervical, prostate, and lung, at the least), should include the entire pertinent sub-populations (as suggested by current guidelines), and should be stated in 2020 dollars, it is clear that aggregate cancer screening costs in the United States currently run in the billions of dollars. Inclusion of all pertinent screening/early detection costs would push total projected direct medical costs for cancer in 2020 from $173 billion toward $200 billion—precisely by how much remains to be determined. The same general conclusion holds for the national-level costs of primary prevention activities undertaken by individuals (for which there are no aggregate estimates at the moment).

The indirect costs of cancer comprise both mortality costs (the monetized value of lost productivity attributable to cancer-related premature death) and morbidity costs (the value of lost productivity attributable to cancer-related time away from work or inefficiency at work). The mortality costs of cancer for the United States in 2020, based on estimated lost wages among those in the labor force, has been projected at nearly $148 billion (Bradley et al., 2008). In an extension of their base-case model that also included the imputed value of lost productivity with respect to nonmarket activities (caregiving and household work), the corresponding 2020 estimate for total cancer-attributable mortality costs in the United States was about $308 billion (Bradley et al., 2008). Now, if morbidity costs are assumed to be about one-third of mortality costs—in line with calculations done for cardiovascular disease (NHLBI, 2009)—then total cancer-attributable morbidity costs for 2020 would be about $49 billion (that is, $148 billion × 0.33 because the National Heart, Lung, and Blood Institute [NHLBI] analysis was based on mortality costs that included only actual wages lost). The resulting projected mortality plus morbidity costs in the United States for 2020 come to $357 billion ($308 billion + $49 billion).

It can be calculated that government expenditures on research—basic, clinical, translation, and population science—and on field-based program implementation related directly or indirectly to cancer control sums to at least $8 billion annually (using data from the Centers for Disease Control and Prevention [CDC] and the National Institutes of Health).[8] It is much more difficult to estimate the biopharmaceutical-sector investment in cancer control efforts—given the very high failure rates inherent in such high-risk investments for drugs, devices, and vaccines. Based on a recent estimate that the biopharmaceutical industry is investing about $90 billion annually on research and development (R&D) in the United States (PhRMA, 2018) and that approximately one-third of the current product pipeline is cancer related (Lloyd, 2018), a reasonable estimate of total annual R&D spending by industry on cancer is $30 billion. Total annual spending by all cancer-related nonprofits in the United States can be estimated at nearly $3 billion, based on an analysis of total reported

[8] Total spending in connection with CDC's National Center for Chronic Disease Prevention and Health Promotion for 2018 fiscal year was estimated at $1.16 billion (CDC, 2019); this included dollars allocated to the Division of Cancer Prevention and Control (DCPC), to tobacco control efforts, to a range of chronic disease prevention and control activities, and to total spending by the states on cancer prevention and control activities. Total National Institutes of Health spending on "cancer" research (basic, clinical, translational, and population sciences) for 2018 fiscal year was $6.36 billion with an additional $1.03 billion for "cancer genomics," for a total of $7.37 billion (NIH, 2019). The total annual government expenditures on cancer control–related research and outreach by these two agencies sums up to $8.53 billion.

contributions to such nonprofits in 2017 as tracked by one of the nation's major charity assessment organizations.[9] Total spending on workplace wellness programs, aimed at reducing the incidence and consequences of cancers and many other diseases, is estimated to be $8 billion annually (Song and Baicker, 2019). And, with total annual U.S. spending on complementary and alternative medicine (CAM) currently at $34 billion, and with an estimated 12 percent of this being for cancer (John et al., 2016), total CAM spending for cancer could be nearly $4 billion. Based on these calculations, the total annual economic burden of cancer in the United States is nearly $600 billion annually,[10] and could well approach $1 trillion in the years ahead given the escalating incidence of cancer in an aging society and multiple other factors, including behavioral choices.

A 2000 NCI analysis of willingness to pay (WTP) for a life year lost to cancer (Yabroff et al., 2008), which assumed that each life year lost due to cancer was worth $150,000, found a WTP of $960.6 billion (in year 2000 dollars). Recast in 2020 terms, the cost could presumably be more than $1 trillion. Based on economic theory, the WTP method is, in principle, the appropriate approach to discern the decision maker's value for any good or service. But there are important behavioral, informational, and incentive-based challenges in identifying the "true value" of that WTP

[9] Charity Navigator (2019), a nonprofit organization that monitors the performance of philanthropies across the United States, has defined a general category of "Health" nonprofits, which is then broken out into four sub-categories, as listed below. For each subcategory, information is provided here on the total number of nonprofits included, the number that were deemed to be cancer-related by virtue of the brief description submitted for each organization, and the total amount of revenue (in thousands of dollars) reported for 2017 by all the cancer-related organizations in the sub-category. The focus is on total reported revenue under the assumption that over the long term, it serves to establish a ceiling on expenditures. The sub-categories are Diseases, Disorders, and Disciplines (267 nonprofits, and 39 cancer-related with total revenues $1,600,976); Patient and Family Support (308 nonprofits, and 104 cancer-related with total revenues $429,952); Treatment and Prevention Services (229 nonprofits, and 7 cancer-related with total revenues $132,600); and Medical Research (148 nonprofits, 46 cancer-related with total revenues $524,845). Summing across the sub-categories yields about $2.7 billion. Because it is highly likely that some nonprofits that are not expressly cancer-designated provide services or assistance to cancer patients and their families and because all relevant nonprofits in the nation may not be included under the Charity Navigator broad category of "Health," a total annual estimate of $3 billion was regarded as a reasonable upper bound.

[10] This rounded estimate of $600 billion was arrived at by thus summing direct medical cost ($173 billion), indirect (productivity) cost ($357 billion), government research and program implementation ($8 billion), biopharmaceutical-sector investment ($30 billion), spending by cancer-related nonprofits ($3 billion), expenditures on workplace wellness programs (8 billion), and cancer-related CAM expenditures ($4 billion)—totaling to $583 billion. Given that direct medical cost does not include spending on screening/early detection and primary prevention activities by individuals, $600 billion is arguably a conservative upper bound on the current total cost of cancer in the United States.

for health outcomes. As a practical matter, this WTP to avoid disease is not the standard basis for estimating disease burden in the United States or elsewhere.

In health and medical sectors, the cost of care and the financial incentives that can influence prescribing and other care decisions have recently become targets for health care reform efforts and reigning in costs. Participants across the health and medical systems have increasingly advocated for the concept of "high-value care" as a way to move forward on health policy matters, but this raises questions about what constitutes "high value" in cancer control, with "value" left undefined or variously defined. A narrow and commonly used definition for "value" is outcome divided by cost (Porter and Teisberg, 2006). However, outcomes for cancer are multidimensional, at best reducing to perhaps a vector for analysis rather than a single value to be divided by cost. Beyond the obvious important outcome of survival, quality of life, symptom and side effect burden, and even quality of death are important factors. Many outcomes other than survival are not well quantified for benchmarking. Nevertheless, a significant move toward paying for quality and value is under way in cancer care. Even if one knew exactly what constitutes and how best to measure both quality and value, cancer control in the clinical setting remains a multispecialty effort. To whom is an outcome attributed when multiple clinicians are involved in treating a patient's cancer? Even if one could settle on a coherent and consistent definition of value in cancer care, how might one transition care models from a fee-for-service system (i.e., one that pays for quantity of health care procedures and interventions) to one that incentivizes clinicians to pursue "value"? These multifaceted relationships in medical care add to the existing complexity, and incentives are difficult to align because the clinicians may function as agents for patients, payers, and health care organizations (Casalino, 2001; Conrad, 2015).

Despite these uncertainties, the emphasis on "quality metrics" and "alternative payment models" such as bundled payments and accountable care organizations has grown, especially after passage of the Patient Protection and Affordable Care Act. Efforts to stimulate methods of "pay for value" were extended under the Medicare Access and CHIP (Children's Health Insurance Program) Reauthorization Act of 2015, which embedded a penalty–reward system (Merit-Based Incentive Payment System) within the reimbursement scheme for fee-for-service clinicians receiving Medicare payments. The law also encouraged clinicians to adopt alternative payment models. The Centers for Medicare & Medicaid Services (CMS) Oncology Care Model,[11] which "aims to provide higher quality, more

[11] See https://innovation.cms.gov/initiatives/oncology-care (accessed February 15, 2019).

highly coordinated oncology care at the same or lower cost to Medicare," is one such alternative payment model.

In recent years, reimbursement uncertainties for small oncology practices have prompted a high rate of vertical integration, or consolidation of independent practices into hospital systems—indeed, the rate of vertical integration is among the highest rates of all specialties (Nikpay et al., 2018). While one might expect the salaried pay structure that often accompanies those arrangements to blunt any fee-for-service, volume-driven financial motivators, in reality employers often create bonus compensations for clinicians that, at least in part, rest on productivity benchmarks of clinical volume. Salary bonuses may also include new quality metrics—some that change annually—to motivate clinicians to comply with policy changes that seek to shift toward payment for "value" rather than quantity.

A Systems Approach to Cancer Control

Cancer control policies and practices focused on the different components of cancer control continue to evolve as new evidence becomes available. This has inspired participants involved in cancer control to seek better information to guide decision making and practices with systems approaches. As an example, the learning health care system model strives to enable evidence-informed transformations across the cancer control continuum. The goals of a learning health system are to continually collect and use data to systematically integrate new knowledge into care delivery processes and to improve outcomes and motivate greater collaboration among all participants (IOM, 2007, 2013b).

Other conceptual systems frameworks have also been used to assess and improve certain aspects of cancer control efforts across the continuum. The socioecological model, for example, has been applied to identify and understand the challenges to screening and treatment of certain types of cancers in some communities in the United States (Daley et al., 2011). Variations of the socioecological model have also been used to examine the factors contributing to cancer disparities in communities with low-income residents (Paskett et al., 2016; Warnecke et al., 2008). Although these models can be useful in understanding certain aspects of cancer control, they are unable to holistically view cancer control efforts to obtain an overall perspective on the collective behavior of the numerous participants in the ecosystem.

Approaching cancer control as a system of systems would involve an integrated practice of strategies and tactics aimed at helping individuals and society deal with cancer in various ways—by avoiding it in the first place, by detecting it as early as possible, by diagnosing it accurately, by treating it effectively, possibly by managing it as a chronic disease, by addressing the pain and other symptoms caused by the cancer and its treatment, and by addressing current and future costs. This end-to-end approach defines the scope of cancer control for this report. Instructive precedents are available from approaches to infectious diseases in which the concept of "control" as the elimination of disease has over time moved toward "outpacing" the disease and its burden. Such an approach requires the skillful integration of public education, epidemiology, surveillance, prevention, diagnostics, and treatment, reinforced by policy actions and agreements at national and international levels. Most importantly, the infectious disease community has organized its activities as an adaptive and agile framework of capabilities to respond to the shifting dynamics of pathogen evolution (Dowdle, 1998; Heymann, 2014). Cancer control efforts should be no different. Indeed, a systems approach would make it clear that the effects and costs of cancer extend far beyond this health and medical end-to-end scope and that effective cancer control needs to work at multiple levels of society, starting from the individual patient. A national strategic vision for cancer control would therefore necessarily involve technologies and markets beyond those in public health and medicine.

To overcome the limitations of the current systems-based approaches to cancer control, the committee focused on the concept of a "complex adaptive system." This concept is described in more detail in the following sections, but in broadest terms, a complex adaptive system is a system consisting of individual entities that act to advance their own interests at many levels and that interact with one another, modifying their behavior in response to what is happening in the rest of the system.

A cell is an example of a complex adaptive system. It is complex because its functioning depends completely on the interactions among its various components, and it is adaptive because those components modify their behavior according to conditions inside and outside the cell. This complex adaptive nature of cells makes it exceptionally difficult to understand their normal functioning, much less their functioning in a cancerous state, and it also explains why it is hard to predict the effects of a particular intervention on cancerous tissue.

When dealing with living systems with many different interconnected pieces responding to one another, a push on one part of the system—say, a drug that targets a particular molecule in a cancer cell—will trigger reactionary changes in other parts of the system as it seeks to adapt to this new input. And the precise details of the system matter because small initial differences can be magnified through the interactions and emergent behaviors to produce major differences in outcome. Sometimes a detail that does not seem to have a particularly important role to play may actually be a key factor. Thus, a treatment that works well on a cancer in a laboratory animal may not work at all in humans, or a drug that is effective on a cancer in one tissue may not work against a similar cancer in another type of tissue, or a prevention method that is widely embraced in one context may not be appropriate in another.

The U.S. cancer control system is, like cancer itself, a complex adaptive system. Each entity in the system (e.g., in public health or clinical or basic research or palliative care or survivorship services) attempts both to serve its own interests and to provide quality products and services to patients and consumers. The ultimate result, in the broader sense of cancer control, is a vast, interconnected system consisting of many different systems: clinicians, public health professionals, hospitals and other medical facilities, biopharmaceutical and medical device companies, payers, consumer technology and computing firms, research organizations, advocacy and support groups, regulatory agencies, patients and their family members, and so on. In this system, one finds a tremendous number of different plans and approaches for cancer control. There is no central command making decisions and passing orders down through a hierarchical structure to the proper entities, which then carry out the commands. Instead, the various components are mostly independent, each making its own decisions about how best to achieve its goals.

Within the federal government, NCI, CDC, CMS, the Veterans Health Administration, the Environmental Protection Agency, the Department of Defense, and the Department of the Treasury, among many more agencies, all deal with cancer control from their own individual perspectives and with their own individual goals. Each state has developed and implemented its own version of a cancer control plan. Biopharmaceutical, medical device, vaccine, and other technology firms individually research and develop products that can be used in cancer control—and that will make them a profit. Hospitals and medical practices all develop their own approaches (generally informed by national guidelines). Professional societies develop guidelines for best practices in preventing, diagnosing, and treating cancer. Insurance companies set policies for what types of cancer screening and treatment are covered under their plans. There are various degrees of coordination among these entities and approaches but no formal organizational structure.

The result is a system of systems, each chasing its own goals with the tools at its disposal. These individual components are adaptive in the sense that they respond to what is happening around them by changing their behavior so as to give themselves the best chance to meet their own goals. It is a well-acknowledged reality that with no central "control" structure—and, indeed, because the diverse independent agents that make up the cancer control system may resist efforts at reform and may act in ways that actively undermine efforts to move the system in a certain direction—the increasingly specialized and fragmented nature of cancer control efforts debilitates the achievement of greater population health outcomes. This fragmented system enables the continued propagation of well-intentioned but often inadequate decisions and practices that reflect the system's inability to meet the current economic demands and technological capabilities.

In considering cancer control as a complex adaptive system, all these challenges can be understood as the natural outcome of the actions of the various individual agents in the system, each following its own strategies and interacting with other agents. Finding a set of solutions will require a similar comprehensive perspective, and this mind-set defines the foundation, principles, and approach of this report and its recommendations.

Applying a complex adaptive systems approach to cancer control—as a system of systems—would build on current models to support more robust decision making in cancer control by considering the actions and relationships among patients, families, clinicians, researchers, payers, government agencies, policy makers, and for-profit and nonprofit organizations, among others. Table 1-2 summarizes the characteristics of a complex adaptive systems approach and its implications for cancer control.

COMPLEX ADAPTIVE SYSTEMS

As described in the previous sections, the traditional approach to understanding and making changes to cancer control has usually been reductive—one element at a time. This section further examines the nature of complex adaptive systems and how they differ from complicated systems. It begins by first describing the essential difference between the "process" of cancer control and the "system" of cancer control.

"Process" Versus "System"

Throughout the rest of this report, a distinction will be made between the process and the system of cancer control: "process" will refer to what happens and how—that is, to those actions that are taken in cancer control efforts—while "system" will refer to the collection of entities and organizations that carry out the process. Thus, the cancer control continuum depicted in Figure 1-6 is describing the *process* of cancer control, from prevention efforts to diagnosis and treatment to hospice care, while the *system* of cancer control consists of all the health professionals, hospitals and other medical facilities, biopharmaceutical and device companies, payers, consumer technology and computing firms, research

TABLE 1-2 Complex Adaptive Systems Approach and Its Implications for Cancer Control

Complex Adaptive Systems	Implications for Cancer Control
They are *nonlinear and dynamic* and do not inherently reach fixed equilibrium points. As a result, system behaviors may appear to be random or chaotic.	System responses often seem unpredictable and disproportionate to interventions. For example, enormous efforts are often needed to achieve small changes, while at times small improvements in treatment might lead to significant changes in clinical care.
They are composed of *independent agents* whose behaviors are based on physical, psychological, or social rules rather than the demands of system dynamics.	Stakeholders (patients, families, clinicians, suppliers, payers, regulators, etc.) respond based on their perceptions, values, and priorities, which are seldom aligned (e.g., payers might try to constrain short-term costs even when long-term health and economic benefits are easily projected).
Because agents' needs or desires, reflected in their rules, are not homogeneous, their *goals and behaviors are likely to conflict*. In response to these conflicts or competitions, agents tend to adapt to one another's behaviors.	Goals and behaviors of stakeholders often conflict. They may perceive these conflicts and adapt their strategies to counteract their impacts. For example, enormous resources might be devoted to advertising to convince patients of their need for products or services with questionable benefits.
Agents are *intelligent*. As they experiment and gain experience, they learn and change their behaviors accordingly. Thus, overall system behavior inherently changes over time.	As the rules of the system evolve and stakeholders understand the impacts of those rules, they might develop strategies to circumvent these rules, including lobbying to avoid rule changes or to change the rules to their benefit.
Adaptation and learning tend to result in *self-organization*. Behavior patterns emerge rather than being designed into the system. The nature of emergent behaviors may range from valuable innovations to unfortunate accidents.	Stakeholders adapt to the changing environment, learning what works and does not. These behaviors often surprise other stakeholders, who then also need to adapt. For example, industry agents might just pay penalties rather than change behaviors in response to rules in the system.
There is *no single point of control*. System behaviors are often unpredictable and uncontrollable, and no one is "in charge." Consequently, the behaviors of complex adaptive systems can usually be more easily influenced than controlled.	The health care system is a federation of millions of entrepreneurs with no one in charge. No single entity can command change. A portfolio of motivations, incentives, and disincentives is needed but would be difficult to design and deploy, particularly if stakeholders game the process.

organizations, advocacy and support groups, regulatory agencies, and patients and family members that are involved.

An analogy may help to make the distinction clearer. Consider modern car production. In this case, the process would be the manufacture and assembly of the individual pieces into a complete automobile. That assembly could be mapped out with a (very complicated) flowchart indicating what happens to each piece and collection of pieces as they are cut, shaped, welded, screwed, bolted, snapped, sewn, and painted. In speaking about these processes, the focus is on the actions that are taken, not who is carrying out the actions, where they are located, or what their relationships are with the others involved in the process. By contrast, the *system* that carries out automobile production consists of a variety of companies or divisions of companies or individual plants that manufacture the individual components and carry out the assembly of individual parts or of subassemblies.

The efficiency of the system will depend not only on the efficiency of the individual processes but also on how well the various components of the system work in unison. If, for example, the manufacturers of two different parts that were later put together failed to coordinate their efforts, then the parts might not fit together, or they might be made of two or more materials—as in composite airframes—that do not work well together. Thus, anyone who seeks to improve the manufacturing of an automobile must consider not only the processes but also the system in which those processes and standards should function.

The difference between system and process is a distinction that is often overlooked. The cancer control continuum, for example, is sometimes referred to as depicting the system of cancer control rather than the process. This is understandable because the word "system" can be used in both ways—as a collection of components that make up a whole or as a set of rules or procedures for how something is done. To avoid confusion, "system" as used in the remainder of this report, both as an organizing concept and central theme, is a collection of components that constitute a whole. In discussing cancer control, it is important to keep the distinction always in mind because improving a system is a very different challenge than improving processes, with a very different scale of economics.

"Complicated" Versus "Complex"

A key feature of the system of cancer control in the United States relates to its vast and daunting array of different interconnected pieces. Any cursory examination of the system reveals that it is extremely complicated in the sense that it has a large number of components connected in various ways. But it is more than just complicated; it is *complex*. Understanding the difference between the two terms is crucial to understanding the principles and system of cancer control itself.

A classic, if lighthearted, example of a complicated system that is not complex is a Rube Goldberg device. Goldberg, a cartoonist, became famous for his drawings of exceptionally complicated devices that performed simple tasks. A typical Rube Goldberg device would have 20 or 30 elements connected one to another so that, say, flipping a switch at one end set off a series of steps—usually involving a mousetrap and a ball rolling down a chute, among other elements—that culminated in something like dropping a piece of bread into a toaster. The outrageously complicated device was amusing, but it was also very simple, as one could understand its function by looking at each of the steps in turn, thus decomposing the device. Furthermore—and this is a crucial property—a complicated yet "simple" system of this sort can be "optimized" by improving the performance of the individual pieces considered separately, with predictable gains in performance for each change in a component.

Not all systems are quite so simple, however, and not all system design and management problems can be addressed through hierarchical decomposition. In some systems, for example, decomposition may result in the loss of important information about interactions among the system's components. And some systems consist of multiple interacting components where no one is "in charge." That is, they are decentralized systems with no central planner to design and control the system.

Examples of complex adaptive systems include not only ecosystems and living organisms (for which the concept was initially developed) but also national economies, the military–industrial complex, the nation's population health system, and also the cancer control system. Such a system is *adaptive* in the sense that the behavior of the individual entities is not fixed but rather changes over time in ways that are intended to help those entities meet their individual goals. And it is *complex* in that the overall performance of the system cannot be understood in terms of the behavior of the individual entities in isolation but rather is inherently the product of interactions between the different entities, which themselves are constantly changing and adapting to one another.

One straightforward example of a complex adaptive system in practice is the nation's cargo transportation system. It consists of various types of carriers (air, rail, highway, and sea), the customers these carriers serve, unions and other organizations of transportation employees, the corporations that develop and build transportation technology (aircraft, trains, cars and trucks, ships, etc.), the government and private agencies responsible for maintaining the nation's transportation infrastructure, various regulators responsible for transportation safety, and many other components. Again, there is no central agency controlling this system.

Government laws and regulations provide a certain amount of direction, but the overall behavior of the system is the product of many different entities pursuing their own goals and adapting their behavior in response to what is happening in the rest of the system. And again, there are emergent behaviors that are produced through the interactions of the various entities in the system, which cannot be understood by analyzing the components one at a time. A good example is the development of container shipping, which offers a way to ship cargo efficiently when it is to be carried by multiple types of carriers—ship, train, and truck. Similar ideas and complexities exist with mail and parcel delivery services, improved over the past century by the U.S. Postal Service and, in more recent decades, by global courier delivery businesses in synergy with available transportation options. Tools from complexity science and systems engineering have been applied to many other complex adaptive systems such as manufacturing, banking, air traffic control, weather prediction, homeland security, and the Internet, to name a few.

Perhaps the most important thing to note about the complex adaptive system of cancer control is that there is no hierarchical command-and-control structure, with someone at the top making decisions and issuing orders that are followed down the hierarchy; instead, there are multiple entities, each with its own goal and acting in ways that are calculated to advance those goals. Generally speaking, these various entities all agree on the general goal—to reduce the burden of cancer—but they have varying interpretations of exactly what that goal means; they have their own individual approaches, scale, and scope to attaining that goal; and they usually have additional objectives that are not necessarily related to that overarching goal. Oncologists treat the cancers that have been diagnosed in their patients and generally leave cancer prevention to other clinicians and public health professionals. Biopharmaceutical and device companies and for-profit hospitals seek to maximize returns for their shareholders while they are providing treatments for patients with cancer.

In the resulting system of systems, each participant pursues its own goals with the tools it has at its disposal. These individual components are adaptive in the sense that they respond to what is happening around them by changing their behavior so as to give themselves the best chance to meet their own goals. When necessary, the different entities communicate and coordinate with one another, but because there is no central command, there is much less coordination than found in a hierarchical system, and the different entities end up adapting their behavior in response to what other entities in the system are doing. In short, there is no such thing as a simple cause and effect in the nation's system for cancer control, and one cannot understand the system by the traditional approach of breaking it down into its component parts and studying each of those parts. What this means for cancer control is that it is very difficult to "optimize" the performance of the entire system using the traditional command-and-control approach. Even in the best-case scenario, with all the participating entities being well intentioned and acting in ways they judge to be ideal for cancer control, the value generated by the cancer control system will inevitably be much lower than it might be, in the sense that health outcomes may be compromised, disparities may be perpetuated, or the costs of delivering these outcomes may be excessive—or all of these.

Consider, for example, what happens when a new cancer diagnostic tool is introduced into the market (Rouse, 2000). In a simpler system, one whose components can be hierarchically decomposed, the introduction of this new technology would be expected to inevitably lead to improved cancer diagnosis and reduced cancer mortality throughout the entire system. In a complex adaptive system, however, all the entities have their own goals and strategies, and there is no one central command that can send out an order for everyone to do what is necessary to ensure that an effective technology is adopted and used. Instead, there are many different components of the system—regulation, clinical evaluation, public awareness, clinician education, coverage and reimbursement, patient preferences, and advocacy, to name a few—that need to be mobilized to do what is necessary to get the new technology adopted and used, or else the patients may not experience the benefits of the new technology. The result is that, in general, enormous investments in biomedical research will not substantially improve health care outcomes unless they are introduced with an understanding of the roles that the different components of the health and medical system play, including their interactions with one another.

In short, the population health and clinical care system in the United States consists of what might be called a "networks of networks" or "systems of systems" that includes an enormous number of independent—and often conflicting—participants and interests, layered by organizations, specialties, regions, cancer types, and so on. A policy that seeks a particular outcome by changing one component or the behavior of one entity of the system will affect the behavior of the other entities. Therefore, the challenges of cancer control—and of health and medical care in the United States in general—need to be addressed in a different way and from a different point of view, recognizing that cancer control is a complex adaptive system, with all that this implies. Figure 1-7 is a descriptive illustration of cancer control as a complex adaptive system composed of multiple subsystems. It displays the level of complexity imposed on cancer control efforts by a range of interacting biological and environmental factors that drive cancer risk, randomness, emergence, and progression.

With all the complexities in cancer control, ultimately the central question remains: Do various forms of cancer control efforts produce adequate

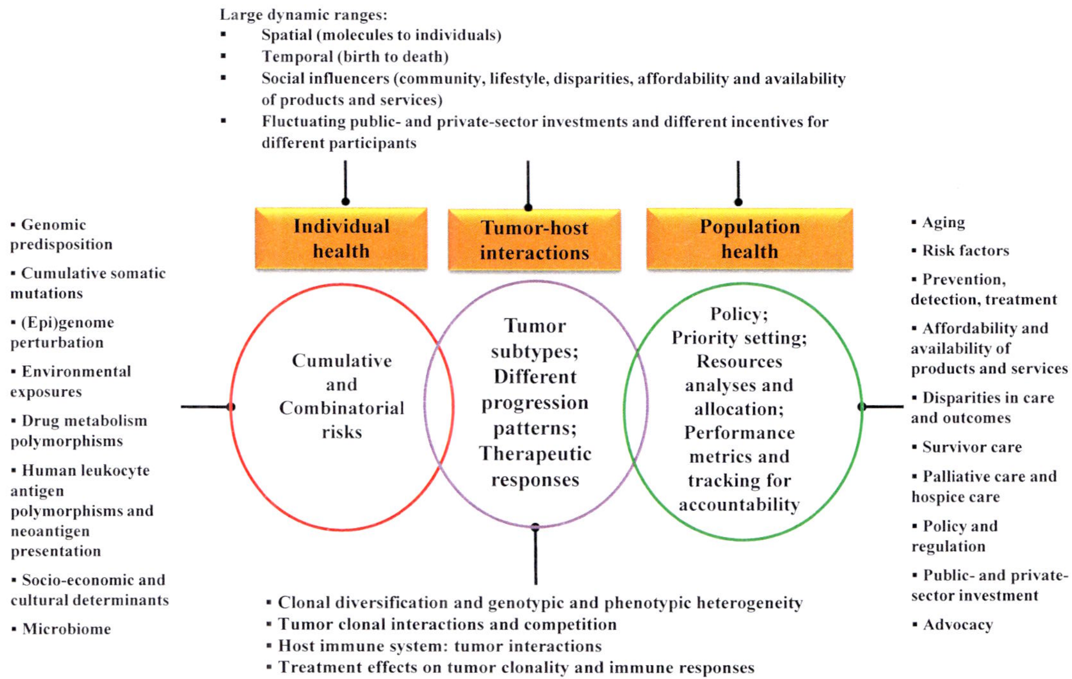

FIGURE 1-7 Cancer control as a complex adaptive system comprising multiple complex adaptive systems and major high-level parameters that contribute to complexity in three domains: individual risk, the complexity of tumor–host interactions in tumor progression, and the complexity of implementation of control efforts across the cancer continuum. Additional levels of complexity are imposed by the large dynamic ranges of the interacting biological and environmental factors and control efforts as well as randomness.

return on public and private investments that are laden with risks? This central question continues to perplex the scientific, business, and policy communities and, ultimately, the taxpayers, as the expenditures in cancer control seem to uncontrollably increase each year. One way to assess the return on the investment would be to consider changes in population health outcomes attributable to cancer prevention and care strategies and to relate these changes to different types of cancer control expenditures. As noted earlier, age-adjusted cancer mortality rates have declined over the past several decades, thanks in part to new cancer screening tests, diagnostics, and treatments as well as to changes in population behaviors that have taken place. But these trends are confounded by simultaneous significant increases in the age-adjusted incidence of some cancers and several other diseases. Because cancer is not one disease, it becomes even more difficult to pinpoint which particular cancer control strategies are driving declines in cancer mortality and in what contexts of care and related services. An objective assessment of the effectiveness and cost of current forms of cancer control efforts would require complex systems analyses.

FINDINGS

Finding 1-1: *Decades of research and development have revealed the intrinsic biological, financial, and social complexities of cancer control. Given the heterogeneity of cancers, it is not always clear whether knowledge and insights gained about one type of cancer can be applied to another type. The growth and metastasis of any type of cancer involve multiple interacting processes, so to gain a complete understanding of that cancer, one needs to comprehend not only the processes but also the ways in which they work with and against one another.*

Finding 1-2: *None of the methods of classifying cancers is sufficient on its own for addressing all the complexities inherent in cancer control.*

Finding 1-3: *Approaching cancer control efforts as if they formed a simple hierarchical "command-and-control" system is inappropriate and ineffective. The outcomes of cancer control in response to a specific change are not generally predictable because of the varied interactions, interests, and influences among its numerous participants. This makes the monitoring of the state and function of the entire "system" of cancer control difficult, especially from an economics perspective and for determining the financial, social, and other returns on investments.*

Finding 1-4: *The total annual economic burden of cancer in the United States is around $600 billion annually and could well approach $1 trillion in the years ahead. It is presently unclear what the current total, including hidden and* *unpriced, costs of cancer control efforts are—from all forms of risk recognition and mitigation to medical treatments and palliative care, supporting research and development, investments across numerous sectors, and other forms of indirect and social expenditures.*

Finding 1-5: *Formidable challenges will continue to exist going forward, not only with respect to essential workforce development for reducing cancer burden and disparities but also in containing the severe financial impacts on patients and their families as well as on public and private payers.*

Finding 1-6: *The cancer control continuum includes activities from recognizing cancer risks to diagnosis and treatment to hospice care, but in practice the sequence of activities is not integrated effectively, with possible adverse consequences for patients, including disparities in outcomes.*

Finding 1-7: *The key differences between the "process" of cancer control and the "system" of cancer control are not widely appreciated. This could negatively affect the coordination needed across the activities and participants in the cancer control continuum.*

Finding 1-8: *A critical intellectual as well as practical challenge arises in determining the "value" of cancer control programs and interventions and how to pay for them. Value considerations are based on wide-ranging interests and perspectives without broad agreement. Cost–effectiveness ratios have been widely used for valuation in health and medical decision making, but they are known to be incomplete.*

Finding 1-9: *As more and more of the genetic, molecular, and biochemical details of cancers are made clear, and as diagnostics, treatments, and combination technologies become sophisticated, clinicians and other professionals are challenged to keep up with the current developments in cancer control and to effectively communicate these advances to patients and their families.*

Finding 1-10: *Differing philosophies can lead to differing policy judgments even in an area that is as seemingly apolitical as cancer control. Some, for example, may believe that the benefits of environmental and workforce programs are outweighed by the costs to businesses and economic competitiveness, while others may see efforts to limit smoking and alcohol consumption and to modify other behaviors as an infringement on individual rights.*

Finding 1-11: *Because outcome measures shape the goals of cancer control programs by implicitly defining what is important for "success," it becomes necessary to critically and accountably analyze which outcomes are most relevant to patients.*

REFERENCES

Abiola, S. E., J. Colgrove, and M. M. Mello. 2013. The politics of HPV vaccination policy formation in the United States. *Journal of Health Politics, Policy and Law* 38(4):645–681.

ACS CAN (American Cancer Society Cancer Action Network). 2017. *The costs of cancer: Addressing patient costs.* https://www.fightcancer.org/sites/default/files/Costs%20of%20Cancer%20-%20Final%20Web.pdf (accessed February 15, 2019).

Ahluwalia, S. C., C. Chen, L. Raaen, A. Motala, A. M. Walling, M. Chamberlin, C. O'Hanlon, J. Larkin, K. Lorenz, O. Akinniranye, and S. Hempel. 2018. A systematic review in support of the national consensus project clinical practice guidelines for quality palliative care, fourth edition. *Journal of Pain and Symptom Management* 56(6):831–870.

Allen, S. I., J. Foulds, E. Wasserman, S. Veldheer, S. Hrabovsky, J. Yingst, and G. Liu. 2018. Tobacco use among middle and high school students in Pennsylvania. *Preventing Chronic Disease* 15:E19.

ASCO (American Society of Clinical Oncology). 2017. The state of cancer care in America, 2017: A report by the American Society of Clinical Oncology. *Journal of Oncology Practice* 13(4):e353–e394.

ASCO. 2018. *National survey reveals surprising number of Americans believe alternative therapies can cure cancer.* https://www.asco.org/advocacy-policy/asco-in-action/national-survey-reveals-surprising-number-americans-believe (accessed February 15, 2019).

Attia, A. C., J. Wolf, and A. E. Núñez. 2018. On surmounting the barriers to HPV vaccination: We can do better. *Annals of Medicine* 50(3):209–225.

Backholer, K., and J. Martin. 2017. Sugar-sweetened beverage tax: The inconvenient truths. *Public Health Nutrition* 20(18):3225–3227.

Banegas, M. P., G. P. Guy, Jr., J. S. de Moor, D. U. Ekwueme, K. S. Virgo, E. E. Kent, S. Nutt, Z. Zheng, R. Rechis, and K. R. Yabroff. 2016. For working-age cancer survivors, medical debt and bankruptcy create financial hardships. *Health Affairs (Millwood)* 35(1):54–61.

Bardia, A., D. L. Barton, L. J. Prokop, B. A. Bauer, and T. J. Moynihan. 2006. Efficacy of complementary and alternative medicine therapies in relieving cancer pain: A systematic review. *Journal of Clinical Oncology* 24(34):5457–5464.

Bernard, D. S., S. L. Farr, and Z. Fang. 2011. National estimates of out-of-pocket health care expenditure burdens among nonelderly adults with cancer: 2001 to 2008. *Journal of Clinical Oncology* 29(20):2821–2826.

Berrigan, D., J. A. Hipp, P. M. Hurvitz, P. James, M. M. Jankowska, J. Kerr, F. Laden, T. Leonard, R. A. McKinnon, T. M. Powell-Wiley, E. Tarlov, and S. N. Zenk. 2015. Geospatial and contextual approaches to energy balance and health. *Annals of GIS* 21(2):157–168.

Bluethmann, S. M., A. B. Mariotto, and J. H. Rowland. 2016. Anticipating the "silver tsunami": Prevalence trajectories and comorbidity burden among older cancer survivors in the United States. *Cancer Epidemiology Biomarkers and Prevention* 25(7):1029–1036.

Booth, S. L., J. F. Sallis, C. Ritenbaugh, J. O. Hill, L. L. Birch, L. D. Frank, K. Glanz, D. A. Himmelgreen, M. Mudd, B. M. Popkin, K. A. Rickard, S. St. Jeor, and N. P. Hays. 2001. Environmental and societal factors affect food choice and physical activity: Rationale, influences, and leverage points. *Nutrition Reviews* 59(3 Pt. 2):S21–S39; discussion S57–S65.

Bowers, D. C., P. C. Nathan, L. Constine, C. Woodman, S. Bhatia, K. Keller, and L. Bashore. 2013. Subsequent neoplasms of the CNS among survivors of childhood cancer: A systematic review. *The Lancet Oncology* 14(8):e321–e328.

Bradley, C. J., K. R. Yabroff, B. Dahman, E. J. Feuer, A. Mariotto, and M. L. Brown. 2008. Productivity costs of cancer mortality in the United States: 2000–2020. *JNCI: Journal of the National Cancer Institute* 100(24):1763–1770.

Breslow, L. 1979. *A history of cancer control in the United States, 1946–1971*. DHEW Publication no. (NIH) 79-1516-9. Washington, DC: U.S. National Cancer Institute, Division of Cancer Control and Rehabilitation.

Brodersen, J., and V. D. Siersma. 2013. Long-term psychosocial consequences of false-positive screening mammography. *The Annals of Family Medicine* 11(2):106–115.

Brown, P., and S. de Graaf. 2013. Considering a future which may not exist: The construction of time and expectations amidst advanced-stage cancer. *Health, Risk & Society* 15(6–7):543–560.

Burg, M. A., G. Adorno, E. D. Lopez, V. Loerzel, K. Stein, C. Wallace, and D. K. Sharma. 2015. Current unmet needs of cancer survivors: Analysis of open-ended responses to the American Cancer Society study of cancer survivors II. *Cancer* 121(4):623–630.

Campo, R. A., J. H. Rowland, M. L. Irwin, P. C. Nathan, E. R. Gritz, and A. Y. Kinney. 2011. Cancer prevention after cancer: Changing the paradigm—a report from the American Society of Preventive Oncology. *Cancer Epidemiology and Prevention Biomarkers* 20(10):2317–2324.

Casalino, L. 2001. Managing uncertainty: Intermediate organizations as triple agents. *Journal of Health Politics, Policy and Law* 26(5):1055–1068.

Cataldo, J. K., S. Dubey, and J. J. Prochaska. 2010. Smoking cessation: An integral part of lung cancer treatment. *Oncology* 78(5–6):289–301.

CDC (Centers for Disease Control and Prevention). 2018a. *Current cigarette smoking among adults in the United States*. https://www.cdc.gov/tobacco/data_statistics/fact_sheets/adult_data/cig_smoking/index.htm (accessed February 15, 2019).

CDC. 2018b. *Smoking is down, but almost 38 million American adults still smoke*. https://www.cdc.gov/media/releases/2018/p0118-smoking-rates-declining.html (accessed February 15, 2019).

CDC. 2019. *National Center for Chronic Disease Prevention and Health Promotion FY 2019 Operating Budget (Dollars in Thousands)*. https://www.cdc.gov/chronicdisease/programs-impact/budget/index.htm (accessed February 15, 2019).

Charity Navigator. 2019. *Charity Categories. Health*. https://www.charitynavigator.org/index.cfm?bay=search.categories&categoryid=5 (accessed February 15, 2019).

Chen, Y., J. Sun, L. C. Huang, H. Xu, and Z. Zhao. 2015. Classification of cancer primary sites using machine learning and somatic mutations. *BioMed Research International* 2015:491502.

Clancy, L. 2014. Reducing lung cancer and other tobacco-related cancers in Europe: Smoking cessation is the key. *The Oncologist* 19(1):16–20.

Claxton, G., L. Levitt, M. Rae, and B. Sawyer. 2018. *Increases in cost-sharing payments continue to outpace wage growth*. https://www.healthsystemtracker.org/brief/increases-in-cost-sharing-payments-have-far-outpaced-wage-growth/#item-start (accessed February 15, 2019).

CMS (Centers for Medicare & Medicaid Services). 2018. *Oncology care model*. https://innovation.cms.gov/initiatives/oncology-care (accessed February 15, 2019).

Cohen, E. E., S. J. LaMonte, N. L. Erb, K. L. Beckman, N. Sadeghi, K. A. Hutcheson, M. D. Stubblefield, D. M. Abbott, P. S. Fisher, K. D. Stein, G. H. Lyman, and M. L. Pratt-Chapman. 2016. American Cancer Society head and neck cancer survivorship care guideline. *CA: A Cancer Journal for Clinicians* 66(3):203–239.

Cohen, S. B. 2014. *The concentration of health care expenditures and related expenses for costly medical conditions, 2012*. October 2014. Statistical Brief #455. Rockville, MD: Agency for Healthcare Research and Quality. https://meps.ahrq.gov/data_files/publications/st455/stat455.pdf (accessed February 15, 2019).

Connor, J. 2017. Alcohol consumption as a cause of cancer. *Addiction* 112(2):222–228.

Conrad, D. A. 2015. The theory of value-based payment incentives and their application to health care. *Health Services Research* 50(Suppl. 2):2057–2089.

Coughlin, S., and P. Keckley. 2013. *Breaking constraints: Can incentives change consumer health choices?* https://www2.deloitte.com/insights/us/en/industry/health-plans/breaking-constraints.html (accessed February 15, 2019).

Cramer, J. D., J. T. Johnson, and M. L. Nilsen. 2018. Pain in head and neck cancer survivors: Prevalence, predictors, and quality-of-life impact. *Otolaryngology–Head and Neck Surgery* 159(5):853–858.

Daley, E., A. Alio, E. H. Anstey, R. Chandler, K. Dyer, and H. Helmy. 2011. Examining barriers to cervical cancer screening and treatment in Florida through a socio-ecological lens. *Journal of Community Health* 36(1):121–131.

Damalas, C. A., and I. G. Eleftherohorinos. 2011. Pesticide exposure, safety issues, and risk assessment indicators. *International Journal of Environmental Research and Public Health* 8(5):1402–1419.

Dieleman, J. L., R. Baral, M. Birger, A. L. Bui, A. Bulchis, A. Chapin, H. Hamavid, C. Horst, E. K. Johnson, and J. Joseph. 2016. US spending on personal health care and public health, 1996–2013. *JAMA* 316(24):2627–2646.

Dorell, C. G., D. Yankey, T. A. Santibanez, and L. E. Markowitz. 2011. Human papillomavirus vaccination series initiation and completion, 2008–2009. *Pediatrics* 128(5):830–839.

Dowdle, W. R. 1998. The principles of disease elimination and eradication. *Bulletin of the World Health Organization* 76(Suppl. 2):22–25.

Edge, S. B., and C. C. Compton. 2010. The American Joint Committee on Cancer: The 7th edition of the AJCC cancer staging manual and the future of TNM. *Annals of Surgical Oncology* 17(6):1471–1474.

El-Jawahri, A., T. W. LeBlanc, L. J. Burns, E. Denzen, C. Meyer, L. W. Mau, E. J. Roeland, W. A. Wood, and E. Petersdorf. 2018. What do transplant physicians think about palliative care? A national survey study. *Cancer* 124(23):4556–4566.

El-Shami, K., K. C. Oeffinger, N. L. Erb, A. Willis, J. K. Bretsch, M. L. Pratt-Chapman, R. S. Cannady, S. L. Wong, J. Rose, A. L. Barbour, K. D. Stein, K. B. Sharpe, D. D. Brooks, and R. L. Cowens-Alvarado. 2015. American Cancer Society colorectal cancer survivorship care guidelines. *CA: A Cancer Journal for Clinicians* 65(6):428–455.

Epstein, R. M., P. R. Duberstein, J. J. Fenton, K. Fiscella, M. Hoerger, D. J. Tancredi, G. Xing, R. Gramling, S. Mohile, P. Franks, P. Kaesberg, S. Plumb, C. S. Cipri, R. L. Street, Jr., C. G. Shields, A. L. Back, P. Butow, A. Walczak, M. Tattersall, A. Venuti, P. Sullivan, M. Robinson, B. Hoh, L. Lewis, and R. L. Kravitz. 2017. Effect of a patient-centered communication intervention on oncologist-patient communication, quality of life, and health care utilization in advanced cancer: The voice randomized clinical trial. *JAMA Oncology* 3(1):92–100.

Ferrell, B. R., J. S. Temel, S. Temin, E. R. Alesi, T. A. Balboni, E. M. Basch, J. I. Firn, J. A. Paice, J. M. Peppercorn, T. Phillips, E. L. Stovall, C. Zimmermann, and T. J. Smith. 2017. Integration of palliative care into standard oncology care: American Society of Clinical Oncology clinical practice guideline update. *Journal of Clinical Oncology* 35(1):96–112.

Foulds, J. 2015. Use of electronic cigarettes by adolescents. *Journal of Adolescent Health* 57(6):569–570.

Frederick, N. N., S. L. Bober, L. Berwick, M. Tower, and L. B. Kenney. 2017. Preparing childhood cancer survivors for transition to adult care: The young adult perspective. *Pediatric Blood & Cancer* 64(10):e26544.

Gaertner, J., W. Siemens, J. J. Meerpohl, G. Antes, C. Meffert, C. Xander, S. Stock, D. Mueller, G. Schwarzer, and G. Becker. 2017. Effect of specialist palliative care services on quality of life in adults with advanced incurable illness in hospital, hospice, or community settings: Systematic review and meta-analysis. *British Medical Journal* 357:j2925.

Gany, F., T. Lee, J. Ramirez, D. Massie, A. Moran, M. Crist, T. McNish, G. Winkel, and J. C. Leng. 2014. Do our patients have enough to eat?: Food insecurity among urban low-income cancer patients. *Journal of Health Care for the Poor and Underserved* 25(3):1153–1168.

Gapstur, S. M., J. M. Drope, E. J. Jacobs, L. R. Teras, M. L. McCullough, C. E. Douglas, A. V. Patel, R. C. Wender, and O. W. Brawley. 2018. A blueprint for the primary prevention of cancer: Targeting established, modifiable risk factors. *CA: A Cancer Journal for Clinicians* 68(6):446–470.

Gibson, A. F., L. D'Cruz, M. Janda, V. L. Beesley, R. E. Neale, and I. J. Rowlands. 2016. Beyond survivorship? A discursive analysis of how people with pancreatic cancer negotiate identity transitions in their health. *Journal of Health Psychology* 21(12):3060–3071.

Gilligan, A. M., D. S. Alberts, D. J. Roe, and G. H. Skrepnek. 2018. Death or debt? National estimates of financial toxicity in persons with newly-diagnosed cancer. *American Journal of Medicine* 131(10):1187–1199.

Glantz, S. A., and E. D. Balbach. 2000. *Tobacco war: Inside the California battles.* Berkeley, CA: University of California Press.

Gonzalez, C. A., and E. Riboli. 2006. Diet and cancer prevention: Where we are, where we are going. *Nutrition and Cancer* 56(2):225–231.

Gordon, L. G., K. M. D. Merollini, A. Lowe, and R. J. Chan. 2017. A systematic review of financial toxicity among cancer survivors: We can't pay the co-pay. *Patient* 10(3):295–309.

Griswold, M. G., N. Fullman, C. Hawley, N. Arian, S. R. Zimsen, H. D. Tymeson, V. Venkateswaran, A. D. Tapp, M. H. Forouzanfar, and J. S. Salama. 2018. Alcohol use and burden for 195 countries and territories, 1990–2016: A systematic analysis for the Global Burden of Disease Study 2016. *The Lancet* 392(10152):1015–1035.

Gross, C. P., J. B. Long, J. S. Ross, M. M. Abu-Khalaf, R. Wang, B. K. Killelea, H. T. Gold, A. B. Chagpar, and X. Ma. 2013. The cost of breast cancer screening in the Medicare population. *JAMA Internal Medicine* 173(3):220–226.

Guadagnolo, B. A., J. Huo, T. A. Buchholz, and D. G. Petereit. 2014. Disparities in hospice utilization among American Indian Medicare beneficiaries dying of cancer. *Ethnicity & Disease* 24(4):393–398.

Guadagnolo, B. A., K. P. Liao, S. H. Giordano, L. S. Elting, and Y. C. Shih. 2015. Variation in intensity and costs of care by payer and race for patients dying of cancer in texas: An analysis of registry-linked Medicaid, Medicare, and dually eligible claims data. *Medical Care* 53(7):591–598.

Guerard, E. J., G. Nightingale, K. Bellizzi, P. Burhenn, A. Rosko, A. S. Artz, B. Korc-Grodzicki, B. Canin, W. Dale, and B. Ferrell. 2016. Survivorship care for older adults with cancer: U13 conference report. *Journal of Geriatric Oncology* 7(4):305–312.

Hagenaars, L. L., P. P. T. Jeurissen, and N. S. Klazinga. 2017. The taxation of unhealthy energy-dense foods (EDFs) and sugar-sweetened beverages (SSBs): An overview of patterns observed in the policy content and policy context of 13 case studies. *Health Policy* 121(8):887–894.

Hall, M. T., K. T. Simms, J. B. Lew, M. A. Smith, J. M. Brotherton, M. Saville, I. H. Frazer, and K. Canfell. 2018. The projected timeframe until cervical cancer elimination in Australia: A modelling study. *Lancet Public Health* 4(1):e19–e27.

Hanna, N. H., and L. H. Einhorn. 2014. Testicular cancer—discoveries and updates. *New England Journal of Medicine* 371(21):2005–2016.

Hardy, D., W. Chan, C. C. Liu, J. N. Cormier, R. Xia, E. Bruera, and X. L. Du. 2011. Racial disparities in the use of hospice services according to geographic residence and socioeconomic status in an elderly cohort with nonsmall cell lung cancer. *Cancer* 117(7):1506–1515.

Heymann, D. L. 2014. *Control of communicable diseases manual,* 20th ed. Washington, DC: American Public Health Association.

Hiatt, R. A., and J. G. Brody. 2018. Environmental determinants of breast cancer. *Annual Review of Public Health* 39:113–133.

Holman, D. M., V. Benard, K. B. Roland, M. Watson, N. Liddon, and S. Stokley. 2014. Barriers to human papillomavirus vaccination among US adolescents: A systematic review of the literature. *JAMA Pediatrics* 168(1):76–82.

Huang, Y., J. Pomeranz, P. Wilde, S. Capewell, T. Gaziano, M. O'Flaherty, R. Kersh, L. Whitsel, D. Mozaffarian, and R. Micha. 2018. Adoption and design of emerging dietary policies to improve cardiometabolic health in the US. *Current Atherosclerosis Reports* 20(5):25.

IARC (International Agency for Research on Cancer) Working Group on the Evaluation of Carcinogenic Risks to Humans. 2007. Meeting, World Health Organization and International Agency for Research on Cancer. *Human papillomaviruses* (Vol. 90). Lyon, France: World Health Organization.

Idikio, H. A. 2011. Human cancer classification: A systems biology-based model integrating morphology, cancer stem cells, proteomics, and genomics. *Journal of Cancer* 2:107–115.

IOM (Institute of Medicine). 1999. *Health effects of exposure to radon: BEIR VI*. Washington, DC: National Academy Press.

IOM. 2002. *Estimating the public health benefits of proposed air pollution regulations*. Washington, DC: The National Academies Press.

IOM. 2003. *Childhood cancer survivorship: Improving care and quality of life*. Washington, DC: The National Academies Press.

IOM. 2006a. *Asbestos: Selected cancers*. Washington, DC: The National Academies Press.

IOM. 2006b. *From cancer patient to cancer survivor: Lost in transition*. Washington, DC: The National Academies Press.

IOM. 2007. *The Learning Healthcare System: Workshop summary*. Washington, DC: The National Academies Press.

IOM. 2008. *Cancer care for the whole patient: Meeting psychosocial health needs*. Washington, DC: National Academies Press.

IOM. 2013a. *Delivering high-quality cancer care: Charting a new course for a system in crisis*. Washington, DC: The National Academies Press.

IOM. 2013b. *Best care at lower cost: The path to continuously learning health care in America*. Washington, DC: The National Academies Press.

IOM. 2015. *Dying in America: Improving quality and honoring individual preferences near the end of life*. Washington, DC: The National Academies Press.

IQVIA Institute for Human Data Science. 2018. *Global oncology trends 2018*. Parsippany, NJ: IQVIA.

Islami, F., A. Goding Sauer, K. D. Miller, R. L. Siegel, S. A. Fedewa, E. J. Jacobs, M. L. McCullough, A. V. Patel, J. Ma, I. Soerjomataram, W. D. Flanders, O. W. Brawley, S. M. Gapstur, and A. Jemal. 2018. Proportion and number of cancer cases and deaths attributable to potentially modifiable risk factors in the United States. *CA: A Cancer Journal for Clinicians* 68(1):31–54.

Israel, B. 2010. *How many cancers are caused by the environment?* https://www.scientificamerican.com/article/how-many-cancers-are-caused-by-the-environment (accessed February 15, 2019).

Jacobs, E. J., C. C. Newton, B. D. Carter, D. Feskanich, N. D. Freedman, R. L. Prentice, and W. D. Flanders. 2015. What proportion of cancer deaths in the contemporary United States is attributable to cigarette smoking? *Annals of Epidemiology* 25(3):179–182.

Jacobsen, P. B., A. P. DeRosa, T. O. Henderson, D. K. Mayer, C. S. Moskowitz, E. D. Paskett, and J. H. Rowland. 2018. Systematic review of the impact of cancer survivorship care plans on health outcomes and health care delivery. *Journal of Clinical Oncology* 36(20):2088–2100.

Jagai, J. S., L. C. Messer, K. M. Rappazzo, C. L. Gray, S. C. Grabich, and D. T. Lobdell. 2017. County-level cumulative environmental quality associated with cancer incidence. *Cancer* 123(15):2901–2908.

Jawerth, N. 2018. Killing more cancer cells than ever before: A new era in radiotherapy. *IAEA Bulletin*. P. 5.

Joffe, M. 2015. *Long-term trends in medicaid spending by the states*. https://www.mercatus.org/system/files/Joffe-State-Medicaid-Spending.pdf (accessed February 15, 2019).

John, G. M., D. L. Hershman, L. Falci, Z. Shi, W.-Y. Tsai, and H. Greenlee. 2016. Complementary and alternative medicine use among US cancer survivors. *Journal of Cancer Survivorship* 10(5):850–864.

Kakushadze, Z., R. Raghubanshi, and W. Yu. 2017. Estimating cost savings from early cancer diagnosis. *Data* 2(3):30.

Kenney, L. B., P. Melvin, L. N. Fishman, J. O'Sullivan-Oliveira, G. S. Sawicki, S. Ziniel, L. Diller, and S. M. Fernandes. 2017. Transition and transfer of childhood cancer survivors to adult care: A national survey of pediatric oncologists. *Pediatric Blood & Cancer* 64(2):346–352.

Kerr, J., C. Anderson, and S. M. Lippman. 2017. Physical activity, sedentary behaviour, diet, and cancer: An update and emerging new evidence. *The Lancet Oncology* 18(8):e457–e471.

KFF (Kaiser Family Foundation). 2017. *How much does the U.S. spend to treat different diseases?* https://www.healthsystemtracker.org/chart-collection/much-u-s-spend-treat-different-diseases/#item-start (accessed February 15, 2019).

Kiadaliri, A. A., J. Jarl, G. Gavriilidis, and U.-G. Gerdtham. 2013. Alcohol drinking cessation and the risk of laryngeal and pharyngeal cancers: A systematic review and meta-analysis. *PLoS ONE* 8(3):e58158.

Kissick, W. L. 1994. *Medicine's dilemmas: Infinite needs versus finite resources*. New Haven, CT: Yale University Press.

Kline, R. M., N. K. Arora, C. J. Bradley, E. R. Brauer, D. L. Graves, N. B. Lunsford, M. S. McCabe, S. F. Nasso, L. Nekhlyudov, J. H. Rowland, R. M. Schear, and P. A. Ganz. 2018. Long-term survivorship care after cancer treatment—summary of a 2017 National Cancer Policy Forum workshop. *Journal of the National Cancer Institute* 110(12):1300–1310.

Koury, J., M. Lucero, C. Cato, L. Chang, J. Geiger, D. Henry, J. Hernandez, F. Hung, P. Kaur, G. Teskey, and A. Tran. 2018. Immunotherapies: Exploiting the immune system for cancer treatment. *Journal of Immunology Research* 2018:9585614.

Kuchenbaecker, K. B., J. L. Hopper, D. R. Barnes, K.-A. Phillips, T. M. Mooij, M.-J. Roos-Blom, S. Jervis, F. E. Van Leeuwen, R. L. Milne, and N. Andrieu. 2017. Risks of breast, ovarian, and contralateral breast cancer for BRCA1 and BRCA2 mutation carriers. *JAMA* 317(23):2402–2416.

Lathan, C. S., A. Cronin, R. Tucker-Seeley, S. Y. Zafar, J. Z. Ayanian, and D. Schrag. 2016. Association of financial strain with symptom burden and quality of life for patients with lung or colorectal cancer. *Journal of Clinical Oncology* 34(15):1732–1740.

Lehman, E. P. 2015. The health care "iron triangle" and the patient protection and Affordable Care Act. *Cleveland Clinic Journal of Medicine* 82(2):73–80.

Li, C. 2012. *Biomarkers to distinguish aggressive cancers from non-aggressive or non-progressing cancer*. https://edrn.nci.nih.gov/protocols/362-biomarkers-to-distinguish-aggressive-cancers-from (accessed February 15, 2019).

Liu, C., Y. Yang, and Y. Wu. 2018. Recent advances in exosomal protein detection via liquid biopsy biosensors for cancer screening, diagnosis, and prognosis. *AAPS Journal* 20(2):41.

Liu, G., E. Wasserman, L. Kong, and J. Foulds. 2017. A comparison of nicotine dependence among exclusive e-cigarette and cigarette users in the path study. *Preventive Medicine* 104:86–91.

Lloyd, I. *Pharma R&D Annual Review 2018.* https://pharmaintelligence.informa.com/resources/product-content/pharma-rd-annual-review-2018 (accessed February 15, 2019).

Lobb, E. A., J. Lacey, J. Kearsley, W. Liauw, L. White, and A. Hosie. 2015. Living with advanced cancer and an uncertain disease trajectory: An emerging patient population in palliative care? *BMJ Supportive & Palliative Care* 5(4):352–357.

LoConte, N. K., A. M. Brewster, J. S. Kaur, J. K. Merrill, and A. J. Alberg. 2018. Alcohol and cancer: A statement of the American Society of Clinical Oncology. *Journal of Clinical Oncology* 36(1):83–93.

Lortet-Tieulent, J., A. Goding Sauer, R. L. Siegel, K. D. Miller, F. Islami, S. A. Fedewa, E. J. Jacobs, and A. Jemal. 2016. State-level cancer mortality attributable to cigarette smoking in the United States. *JAMA Internal Medicine* 176(12):1792–1798.

Lowy, D. R., and J. T. Schiller. 2012. Reducing HPV-associated cancer globally. *Cancer Prevention Research* 5(1):18–23.

Lunze, K., and M. K. Paasche-Orlow. 2013. Financial incentives for healthy behavior: Ethical safeguards for behavioral economics. *American Journal of Preventive Medicine* 44(6):659–665.

Mariotto, A. B., K. Robin Yabroff, Y. Shao, E. J. Feuer, and M. L. Brown. 2011. Projections of the cost of cancer care in the United States: 2010–2020. *Journal of the National Cancer Institute* 103(2):117–128.

Martin, A. B., M. Hartman, J. Benson, and A. Catlin. 2016. National health spending in 2014: Faster growth driven by coverage expansion and prescription drug spending. *Health Affairs* 35(1):150–160.

Martinez, M. E., J. R. Marshall, and E. Giovannucci. 2008. Diet and cancer prevention: The roles of observation and experimentation. *Nature Reviews Cancer* 8(9):694–703.

Marzorati, C., S. Riva, and G. Pravettoni. 2017. Who is a cancer survivor? A systematic review of published definitions. *Journal of Cancer Education* 32(2):228–237.

Mayne, S. T., M. C. Playdon, and C. L. Rock. 2016. Diet, nutrition, and cancer: Past, present and future. *Nature Reviews Clinical Oncology* 13(8):504.

McCullough, M. L., and E. L. Giovannucci. 2004. Diet and cancer prevention. *Oncogene* 23(38):6349–6364.

Meeker, C. R., D. M. Geynisman, B. L. Egleston, M. J. Hall, K. Y. Mechanic, M. Bilusic, E. R. Plimack, L. P. Martin, M. von Mehren, B. Lewis, and Y. N. Wong. 2016. Relationships among financial distress, emotional distress, and overall distress in insured patients with cancer. *Journal of Oncology Practice* 12(7):e755–e764.

Méndez, D., O. Alshanqeety, K. E. Warner, P. M. Lantz, and P. N. Courant. 2011. The impact of declining smoking on radon-related lung cancer in the United States. *American Journal of Public Health* 101(2):310–314.

Miller, K. D., R. L. Siegel, C. C. Lin, A. B. Mariotto, J. L. Kramer, J. H. Rowland, K. D. Stein, R. Alteri, and A. Jemal. 2016. Cancer treatment and survivorship statistics, 2016. *CA: A Cancer Journal for Clinicians* 66(4):271–289.

NASEM (National Academies of Sciences, Engineering, and Medicine). 2017. *Driving action and progress on obesity prevention and treatment: Proceedings of a workshop.* Washington DC: The National Academies Press.

NASEM. 2018a. *Making medicines affordable: A national imperative.* Washington, DC: The National Academies Press.

NASEM. 2018b. *Public health consequences of e-cigarettes.* Washington, DC: The National Academies Press.

NCCIH (National Center for Complementary and Integrative Health). 2018. *The use of complementary and alternative medicine in the United States: Cost data.* https://nccih.nih.gov/news/camstats/costs/costdatafs.htm (accessed February 15, 2019).

NCCN (National Comprehensive Cancer Network). 2018. *Survivorship guidelines.* http://www.nccn.org/professionals/physician_gls/default.aspx#survivorship (accessed February 15, 2019).

NCHPC (National Coalition for Hospice and Palliative Care). 2018. *Clinical practice guidelines for quality palliative care*, 4th ed. Richmond, VA: National Coalition for Hospice and Palliative Care.

NCI (National Cancer Institute). 2018a. *Cancer control continuum.* https://cancercontrol.cancer.gov/od/continuum.html (accessed February 15, 2019).

NCI. 2018b. *Cancer facts & the war on cancer.* https://training.seer.cancer.gov/disease/war (accessed February 15, 2019).

NCI. 2018c. *National Cancer Act of 1937.* https://www.cancer.gov/about-nci/legislative/history/national-cancer-act-1937 (accessed February 15, 2019).

NCI. 2019. Definitions. Survivorship. https://cancercontrol.cancer.gov/ocs/statistics/definitions.html (accessed February 15, 2019).

NHLBI (National Heart, Lung, and Blood Institute). 2009. *NHLBI fact book fiscal year 2008.* Bethesda, MD. https://www.nhlbi.nih.gov/files/docs/factbook/FactBook2008.pdf (accessed February 15, 2019).

NIH (National Institutes of Health). 2018. *Fact sheets—cancer.* https://report.nih.gov/nihfactsheets/viewfactsheet.aspx?csid=75 (accessed February 15, 2019).

NIH. 2019. *Estimates of funding for various research, condition, and disease categories.* https://report.nih.gov/categorical_spending.aspx (accessed February 15, 2019).

Nikpay, S. S., M. R. Richards, and D. Penson. 2018. Hospital-physician consolidation accelerated in the past decade in cardiology, oncology. *Health Affairs* 37(7):1123–1127.

O'Donoghue, C., M. Eklund, E. M. Ozanne, and L. J. Esserman. 2014. Aggregate cost of mammography screening in the United States: Comparison of current practice and advocated guidelines. *Annals of Internal Medicine* 160(3):145–153.

O'Dowd, E. L., and D. R. Baldwin. 2017. Lung cancer screening—low dose CT for lung cancer screening: Recent trial results and next steps. *The British Journal of Radiology* 90(1079):20170460.

Ogilvie, G. S., F. Phan, H. N. Pedersen, S. R. Dobson, M. Naus, and E. M. Saewyc. 2018. Population-level sexual behaviours in adolescent girls before and after introduction of the human papillomavirus vaccine (2003–2013). *Canadian Medical Association Journal* 190(41):E1221–E1226.

Olstad, D. L., R. Ancilotto, M. Teychenne, L. M. Minaker, D. R. Taber, K. D. Raine, C. I. J. Nykiforuk, and K. Ball. 2017. Can targeted policies reduce obesity and improve obesity-related behaviours in socioeconomically disadvantaged populations? A systematic review. *Obesity Reviews* 18(7):791–807.

Owen, N., G. N. Healy, C. E. Matthews, and D. W. Dunstan. 2010. Too much sitting: The population health science of sedentary behavior. *Exercise and Sport Sciences Reviews* 38(3):105–113.

Paskett, E., B. Thompson, A. S. Ammerman, A. N. Ortega, J. Marsteller, and D. Richardson. 2016. Multilevel interventions to address health disparities show promise in improving population health. *Health Affairs* 35(8):1429–1434.

PCP (President's Cancer Panel). 2010. *Reducing environmental cancer risk: What we can do now.* https://deainfo.nci.nih.gov/advisory/pcp/annualreports/pcp08-09rpt/pcp_report_08-09_508.pdf (accessed February 15, 2019).

PCP. 2018. *HPV vaccination for cancer prevention: Progress, opportunities, and a renewed call to action: A report to the president of the United States from the chair of the President's Cancer Panel.* https://prescancerpanel.cancer.gov/report/hpvupdate/pdf/PresCancerPanel_HPVUpdate_Nov2018.pdf (accessed February 15, 2019).

PhRMA (Pharmaceutical Research and Manufacturers of America). 2018. *2018 Profile: Biopharmaceutical research industry*. http://phrma-docs.phrma.org/industryprofile/2018/pdfs/2018_IndustryProfile_Brochure.pdf (accessed February 15, 2019).

Pollack, L. A., W. Adamache, A. B. Ryerson, C. R. Eheman, and L. C. Richardson. 2009. Care of long-term cancer survivors: Physicians seen by medicare enrollees surviving longer than 5 years. *Cancer* 115(22):5284–5295.

Porter, M. E., and E. O. Teisberg. 2006. *Redefining health care: Creating value-based competition on results*. Boston, MA: Harvard Business Press.

Prigerson, H. G., Y. Bao, M. A. Shah, M. E. Paulk, T. W. LeBlanc, B. J. Schneider, M. M. Garrido, M. C. Reid, D. A. Berlin, K. B. Adelson, A. I. Neugut, and P. K. Maciejewski. 2015. Chemotherapy use, performance status, and quality of life at the end of life. *JAMA Oncology* 1(6):778–784.

Pruss-Ustun, A., J. Wolf, C. Corvalan, T. Neville, R. Bos, and M. Neira. 2017. Diseases due to unhealthy environments: An updated estimate of the global burden of disease attributable to environmental determinants of health. *Journal of Public Health* 39(3):464–475.

Reuben, S. H. 2010. *Reducing environmental cancer risk: What we can do now. 2008–2009 Annual Report, President's Cancer Panel*. https://deainfo.nci.nih.gov/advisory/pcp/annualreports/pcp08-09rpt/pcp_report_08-09_508.pdf (accessed February 15, 2019).

Riedel, R. F., K. Slusser, S. Power, C. A. Jones, T. W. LeBlanc, A. H. Kamal, D. Desai, D. Allen, Y. Yu, S. Wolf, and A. N. Galanos. 2017. Improvements in patient and health system outcomes using an integrated oncology and palliative medicine approach on a solid tumor inpatient service. *Journal of Oncology Practice* 13(9):e738–e748.

Riley, G. F., A. L. Potosky, C. N. Klabunde, J. L. Warren, and R. Ballard-Barbash. 1999. Stage at diagnosis and treatment patterns among older women with breast cancer: An HMO and fee-for-service comparison. *JAMA* 281(8):720–726.

Rosenberg, S. A., and N. P. Restifo. 2015. Adoptive cell transfer as personalized immunotherapy for human cancer. *Science* 348(6230):62–68.

Rosenthal, E. T., B. Evans, J. Kidd, K. Brown, H. Gorringe, M. van Orman, and S. Manley. 2017. Increased identification of candidates for high-risk breast cancer screening through expanded genetic testing. *Journal of the American College of Radiology* 14(4):561–568.

Rouse, W. B. 2000. Managing complexity: Disease control as a complex adaptive system. *Information-Knowledge-Systems Management* 2(2):143–165.

Rubinstein, E. B., W. L. Miller, S. V. Hudson, J. Howard, D. O'Malley, J. Tsui, H. S. Lee, A. Bator, and B. F. Crabtree. 2017. Cancer survivorship care in advanced primary care practices: A qualitative study of challenges and opportunities. *JAMA Internal Medicine* 177(12):1726–1732.

Runowicz, C. D., C. R. Leach, N. L. Henry, K. S. Henry, H. T. Mackey, R. L. Cowens-Alvarado, R. S. Cannady, M. L. Pratt-Chapman, S. B. Edge, L. A. Jacobs, A. Hurria, L. B. Marks, S. J. LaMonte, E. Warner, G. H. Lyman, and P. A. Ganz. 2016. American Cancer Society/American Society of Clinical Oncology breast cancer survivorship care guideline. *Journal of Clinical Oncology* 34(6):611–635.

Sallis, J. F., R. B. Cervero, W. Ascher, K. A. Henderson, M. K. Kraft, and J. Kerr. 2006. An ecological approach to creating active living communities. *Annual Review of Public Health* 27:297–322.

Siegel, R. L., A. Jemal, R. C. Wender, T. Gansler, J. Ma, and O. W. Brawley. 2018. An assessment of progress in cancer control. *CA: A Cancer Journal for Clinicians* 68(5):329–339.

Siegel, R. L., K. D. Miller, and A. Jemal. 2019. Cancer statistics, 2019. *CA: A Cancer Journal for Clinicians* 69(1):7.

Singh, T., R. A. Arrazola, C. G. Corey, C. G. Husten, L. J. Neff, D. M. Homa, and B. A. King. 2016. Tobacco use among middle and high school students—United States, 2011–2015. *Morbidity and Mortality Weekly Report* 65(14):361–367.

Skolarus, T. A., A. M. Wolf, N. L. Erb, D. D. Brooks, B. M. Rivers, W. Underwood III, A. L. Salner, M. J. Zelefsky, J. B. Aragon Ching, and S. F. Slovin. 2014. American Cancer Society prostate cancer survivorship care guidelines. *CA: A Cancer Journal for Clinicians* 64(4):225–249.

Smith, B. D., G. L. Smith, A. Hurria, G. N. Hortobagyi, and T. A. Buchholz. 2009. Future of cancer incidence in the United States: Burdens upon an aging, changing nation. *Journal of Clinical Oncology* 27(17):2758–2765.

Smith, R. A., K. S. Andrews, D. Brooks, S. A. Fedewa, D. Manassaram-Baptiste, D. Saslow, O. W. Brawley, and R. C. Wender. 2018. Cancer screening in the United States, 2018: A review of current American Cancer Society guidelines and current issues in cancer screening. *CA: A Cancer Journal for Clinicians* 68(4):297–316.

Snyderman, R., and A. T. Weil. 2002. Integrative medicine: Bringing medicine back to its roots. *Archives of Internal Medicine* 162(4):395–397.

Song, Q., S. D. Merajver, and J. Z. Li. 2015. Cancer classification in the genomic era: Five contemporary problems. *Human Genomics* 9:27.

Song, Z., and K. Baicker. 2019. Effect of a workplace wellness program on employee health and economic outcomes: A randomized clinical trial. *JAMA* 321(15):1491–1501.

Soni, A., L. M. Sabik, K. Simon, and B. D. Sommers. 2018. Changes in insurance coverage among cancer patients under the Affordable Care Act. *JAMA Oncology* 4(1):122–124.

Spallarossa, P., G. Meliota, C. Brunelli, E. Arboscello, P. Ameri, C. C. Dessalvi, F. Grossi, M. Deidda, D. Mele, and M. Sarocchi. 2018. Potential cardiac risk of immune-checkpoint blockade as anticancer treatment: What we know, what we do not know, and what we can do to prevent adverse effects. *Medicinal Research Reviews* 38(5):1447–1468.

Stange, K. C., E. S. Breslau, A. J. Dietrich, and R. E. Glasgow. 2012. State-of-the-art and future directions in multilevel interventions across the cancer control continuum. *Journal of the National Cancer Institute Monographs* 2012(44):20–31.

Steward, W., and K. Brown. 2013. Cancer chemoprevention: A rapidly evolving field. *British Journal of Cancer* 109(1):1.

Sudhakar, A. 2009. History of cancer, ancient and modern treatment methods. *Journal of Cancer Science and Therapy* 1(2):1–4.

Thom, B., A. H. Boekhout, S. Corcoran, R. Adsuar, K. C. Oeffinger, and M. S. McCabe. 2019. Advanced practice providers and survivorship care: They can deliver. *Journal of Oncology Practice* 15(3):e230–e237.

Wang, S. Y., J. Hall, C. E. Pollack, K. Adelson, A. J. Davidoff, J. B. Long, and C. P. Gross. 2016. Associations between end-of-life cancer care patterns and medicare expenditures. *Journal of the National Comprehensive Cancer Network* 14(8):1001–1008.

Warnecke, R. B., A. Oh, N. Breen, S. Gehlert, E. Paskett, K. L. Tucker, N. Lurie, T. Rebbeck, J. Goodwin, and J. Flack. 2008. Approaching health disparities from a population perspective: The National Institutes of Health Centers for Population Health and Health Disparities. *American Journal of Public Health* 98(9):1608–1615.

WCRF/AICR (World Cancer Research Fund/American Institute for Cancer Research). 2018. *Diet, nutrition, physical activity and cancer: A global perspective.* Continuous Update Project Expert Report 2018. https://www.wcrf.org/sites/default/files/Summary-third-expert-report.pdf (accessed February 15, 2019).

Welch, H. G., P. C. Prorok, A. J. O'Malley, and B. S. Kramer. 2016. Breast-cancer tumor size, overdiagnosis, and mammography screening effectiveness. *New England Journal of Medicine* 375(15):1438–1447.

White, M. C., F. Babcock, N. S. Hayes, A. B. Mariotto, F. L. Wong, B. A. Kohler, and H. K. Weir. 2017. The history and use of cancer registry data by public health cancer control programs in the United States. *Cancer* 123(Suppl. 24):4969–4976.

Wright, A. A., B. Zhang, A. Ray, J. W. Mack, E. Trice, T. Balboni, S. L. Mitchell, V. A. Jackson, S. D. Block, P. K. Maciejewski, and H. G. Prigerson. 2008. Associations between end-of-life discussions, patient mental health, medical care near death, and caregiver bereavement adjustment. *JAMA* 300(14):1665–1673.

Yabroff, K. R., C. J. Bradley, A. B. Mariotto, M. L. Brown, and E. J. Feuer. 2008. Estimates and projections of value of life lost from cancer deaths in the United States. *JNCI: Journal of the National Cancer Institute* 100(24):1755–1762.

Zhang, B., A. A. Wright, H. A. Huskamp, M. E. Nilsson, M. L. Maciejewski, C. C. Earle, S. D. Block, P. K. Maciejewski, and H. G. Prigerson. 2009. Health care costs in the last week of life: Associations with end-of-life conversations. *Archives of Internal Medicine* 169(5):480–488.

2

The Current "System" of Cancer Control

The cancer control efforts of the United States are remarkably complex, and there have been many successes and setbacks. The system has evolved over time in a mostly undesigned way, with no overarching strategy or guiding vision of what an ideal cancer control system should operate or perform. The system is the product of hundreds of independent or near-autonomous cancer control efforts—research into the biology and epidemiology of cancer, improvements in surgery or radiation therapy, diagnostic and other product engineering, drug development and testing, hospice care, payment and reimbursement policies, and on and on. On various occasions, some organization, usually a government agency or professional group, has attempted to impose some sort of post hoc structure and direction on this system—such as by developing a "national cancer plan"—and to increase collaboration and coordination among the system's various components. But, for the most part, the system still remains reactive with a near-term focus.

This chapter offers a brief overview of cancer control efforts pursued by different groups within the United States and around the world. The picture that emerges of the U.S. cancer control system is an amalgam of independent entities each possibly working toward a common goal but often not following a common strategic vision, with relatively little collaboration and cooperation with one another and with no overarching strategy that sets forth how these different components should be working together on cancer control.

GLOBAL EFFORTS IN CANCER CONTROL

Eighty-two percent of World Health Organization (WHO) member countries (158 nations) have established some form of high-level guidance system for cancer control, and these systems vary greatly according to the needs of their populations (Romero et al., 2018). The United Kingdom's plan, for instance, places more emphasis on cancer prevention and survivorship care. Germany's national plan prioritizes improving the early detection of cancers, increasing cancer care effectiveness and quality, and empowering patients within the medical system. Malaysia has recognized both conventional and complementary medicine for cancer control and has developed specific targets as part of its strategies for noncommunicable diseases (NCDs). Australia's plan has centered on identifying effective indicators and standards for performance evaluation across all areas of cancer control. Canada's recent plan has set milestones for cancer control subject to routine evaluations for a 30-year period. Peru's cancer control plan has focused on expanding national funding within its public health system and providing universal health coverage for cancer care to the most vulnerable populations.

Japan's plan for cancer control has prioritized improvements in clinical services, facilities, and registries as well as in related biomedical research (Hanyuda, 2012). China's plan is designed to improve cancer registries, prioritize human papillomavirus (HPV) vaccine research and development, and advance the use of traditional medicines for prevention and treatment (Economist Intelligence Unit, 2015). India, the developer of one of the earliest national cancer control plans, has recently focused on establishing pain relief and palliative care networks throughout the subcontinent (Rath and Gandhi, 2014).

About 7.3 percent of total worldwide cancer deaths have been reported to occur in Africa (Bray et al., 2018). The various plans of African nations commonly include policies to curb tobacco use by taxation, raising the minimum age for purchase, and restricting related product marketing and advertising. As examples, Kenya's recent plan has focused on improving cancer registries and surveillance practice, in addition to involving non–health sector participants in cancer control (Kenya Ministry of Health, 2017), and Rwanda's national plan has focused on universal HPV vaccination coverage (Stefan et al., 2013). Table 2-1 provides a glimpse of the variation in all the countries with national plans for cancer control. Only about half of these national plans include an implementation strategy.

WHO and other agencies of the United Nations have issued a series of reports and resolutions describing the global threat of cancers and proposing ways to reduce the associated risks and burden. In 2005, WHO

TABLE 2-1 Proportion of Countries (n = 158) That Address Elements of Cancer Prevention and Control in Cancer-Related Plans, by Type of Plan

	Physical Activity	Alcohol Consumption	Obesity	Tobacco*	Monitoring	Cost
Any plan (n = 158)						
Not mentioned	13/150 (9%)	21/151 (14%)	22/152 (14%)	16/157 (10%)	32/150 (21%)	89/154 (58%)
Mentioned but without strategy	67/150 (45%)	61/151 (40%)	71/152 (47%)	NA	107/150 (71%)	49/154 (32%)
Mentioned with implementation strategy	70/150 (47%)	69/151 (46%)	59/152 (39%)	141/157 (90%)	11/150 (7%)	16/154 (10%)
NCD plan only (n = 64)						
Not mentioned	7/64 (11%)	7/64 (11%)	12/64 (19%)	10/64 (16%)	13/63 (21%)	37/64 (58%)
Mentioned but without strategy	28/64 (44%)	28/64 (44%)	31/64 (48%)	NA	47/63 (75%)	21/64 (33%)
Mentioned with implementation strategy	29/64 (45%)	29/64 (45%)	21/64 (33%)	54/64 (84%)	3/63 (5%)	6/64 (9%)
NCD plan plus NCCP (n = 65)						
Not mentioned	1/57 (2%)	6/58 (10%)	4/59 (7%)	1/64 (2%)	10/58 (17%)	35/61 (57%)
Mentioned but without strategy	26/57 (46%)	22/58 (38%)	28/59 (47%)	NA	44/58 (76%)	18/61 (30%)
Mentioned with implementation strategy	30/57 (53%)	30/58 (52%)	27/59 (46%)	63/64 (98%)	4/58 (7%)	8/61 (13%)

continued

TABLE 2-1 Continued

	Physical Activity	Alcohol Consumption	Obesity	Tobacco*	Monitoring	Cost
NCCP only (n = 27)						
Not mentioned	5/27 (19%)	6/27 (22%)	6/27 (22%)	3/27 (11%)	8/27 (30%)	15/27 (56%)
Mentioned but without strategy	11/27 (41%)	11/27 (41%)	12/27 (44%)	NA	15/27 (56%)	10/27 (37%)
Mentioned with implementation strategy	11/27 (41%)	10/27 (37%)	9/27 (33%)	24/27 (89%)	4/27 (15%)	2/27 (7%)

NOTES: NA = not applicable; NCCP = national cancer control plan; NCD = noncommunicable disease; Data for two countries that had plans other than NCD plans or NCCPs are not shown here; * For the policy relevance of tobacco as a risk factor for cancer, the questionnaire addressed whether or not a strategy for tobacco control was mentioned.
SOURCE: Table 1 in Romero et al., 2018.

passed a resolution on cancer prevention and control that urged member countries to create national plans to intensify their cancer control efforts. In 2013, WHO's *Global Action Plan for the Prevention and Control of NCDs* gave an extra boost to cancer control efforts—as well as control efforts for other top NCDs such as cardiovascular diseases, chronic respiratory diseases, and diabetes—by setting the target of a 25 percent reduction in premature deaths resulting from NCDs by 2025 (WHO, 2013). That same year, the United Nations Development Programme launched an action plan against NCDs, including cancers. This action plan recognized NCDs as a significant challenge that impedes social and economic development (UNDP, 2013). Two years earlier, after pointing to the "growing danger" and "deepening crisis" of NCDs, the World Bank offered its own recommendations for reducing the rates of cancer, emphasizing increased taxation on tobacco products and providing subsidies for healthier food options (World Bank, 2011).

In another resolution issued at the 2017 World Health Assembly, the United States and other member countries, recognizing the urgent and more serious need to multiply efforts against cancer, adopted an "integrated approach" for cancer control (WHO, 2017), this time directly recognizing the core issues of affordability and availability of cancer interventions (UN, 2017).

FEDERAL EFFORTS IN THE UNITED STATES

Across the U.S. government, cancer control efforts are situated in a wide range of agencies, reflecting the very broad nature of cancer control. Within the Department of Health and Human Services, the lead agency with numerous constituent units interested in cancer, the Centers for Disease Control and Prevention (CDC), the Centers for Medicare & Medicaid Services (CMS), and the National Institutes of Health (NIH) warrant particular mention.

NIH has been a predominant funder and conductor of research and development related to cancer biology, prevention, detection, diagnosis, and treatment, especially through its National Cancer Institute (NCI),[1] while CDC's focus has been to "develop, implement, and promote effective cancer prevention and control practices" (CDC, 2018a) in conjunction with state health agencies, territories, and tribes and tribal organizations. CMS manages the federally funded health insurance programs

[1] A section of the National Cancer Act of 1971 authorized NCI to establish a national cancer program in cooperation with states and health agencies. The NCI director was to coordinate not only the cancer research programs within NCI but also all cancer control efforts related to other federal and nonfederal programs.

that provide coverage to millions of Americans, including those who are 65 years or older, eligible low-income families and children, pregnant women, and people with disabilities.

In addition to NCI, CDC, and CMS, there are a dozen more agencies within HHS whose research, policies, and programs are pertinent to cancer control. The Food and Drug Administration reviews drugs, biologics, and devices for cancer diagnostics and treatment (FDA, 2018). The Office of Population Affairs administers the Title X program on population health, including a program for breast and cervical cancer screening and prevention (HHS, 2018). The Health Resources and Services Administration coordinates the National Center for Health Workforce Analysis, which collects workforce data, develops tools for projecting workforce supply and demand, and evaluates workforce policies and programs (HRSA, 2019). The agency also oversees several cancer-relevant federal programs and initiatives, including the 340B drug discount program.[2] The Agency for Healthcare Research and Quality performs and funds research to improve the quality, safety, efficiency, and effectiveness of medical services and makes those findings publicly available (AHRQ, 2019). The Indian Health Service ensures that culturally appropriate cancer services and surveillance are available and accessible to American Indian and Alaskan Natives to reduce health disparities and ultimately reduce cancer burden (IHS, 2019).[3]

The Department of Veterans Affairs (VA) has conducted cancer research since 1932 (before NCI even existed), when it established its first tumor research laboratory. Recent census data indicate that there are nearly 18.2 million veterans of military service in the United States, half of them over 65 years of age (Census Bureau, 2018). VA provides medical care for approximately 3 percent of U.S. cancer cases each year through the Veterans Health Administration (Zullig et al., 2017). Through the Million Veteran Program, launched in 2011, VA has focused its efforts on gaining a better understanding of how genetic and other variations influence cancer risks and burdens among veterans. Furthermore, as a partner in NIH's All of Us, VA has sought to ensure veteran participation in this research program.

Additional federal agencies involved in cancer control are the Department of Defense (DoD), Department of Energy (DOE), Environmental Protection Agency (EPA), Department of Agriculture (USDA), Department of Education (ED), Department of the Treasury, Department of Labor (DOL),

---

[2] The 340B drug discount program was created by Congress in 1992 with the goal of improving patients' access to outpatient medications by allowing hospitals and clinics that serve high volumes of low-income patients to purchase drugs at discounted prices.

[3] This text has been revised since prepublication release.

Department of Housing and Urban Development (HUD), Department of Commerce (DOC), Office of Management and Budget (OMB), Equal Employment Opportunity Commission (EEOC), Social Security Administration (SSA), and Office of Personnel Management (OPM). Brief descriptions of these agencies' activities follow.

DoD has carried out and provided external funding for cancer research through its congressionally directed medical research programs to support members of the military and their beneficiaries (DoD, 2015). In 1992, with congressional funds, DoD started a breast cancer research program, followed 5 years later by a prostate cancer research program. Subsequently, the congressionally directed medical research programs have expanded to include research on lung, kidney, and ovarian cancers. In addition, the Big Mechanism program, launched in 2014 by the Defense Advanced Research Projects Agency, is aimed at developing automated technologies to understand the biology of cancer as well as the complex interactions that lead cells to become cancerous (Cohen, 2015).

DOE and NIH jointly coordinated the Human Genome Project, which helped advance the scientific understanding of human genetic variation and its impact on population health. In 2018 the agency entered into a new partnership with NCI to launch the Joint Design of Advanced Computing Solutions for Cancer, with the intent of accelerating advances in precision oncology and related computing technologies (DOE, 2018).

EPA has set air and water quality standards since the Clean Air Act of 1970 and the Clean Water Act of 1972. The agency has determined the health hazards of chemical contaminants that may be present in the environment. In addition, EPA manages the integrated risk information system, an electronic database that contains information on human health effects from exposure to certain substances in the environment (EPA, 2018). Furthermore, EPA publishes information on the likely carcinogenic effects of exposure to various contaminants and pollutants in the environment.

USDA's principal involvement in cancer control has been to address a range of food safety issues. The agency's responsibilities include ensuring that the nation's commercial supply of meat, poultry, and egg products is safe, healthful, and correctly labeled and packaged (USDA, 2018a). The agency provides statistical information, including agricultural chemical usage data, related to the safety of the U.S. food supply. Also, every 5 years USDA and HHS jointly publish the *Dietary Guidelines for Americans*, which has been used to guide various other federal policies and programs, including the Supplemental Nutrition Assistance Program (USDA, 2018b), which currently serves 42 million people (CBPP, 2018), and the National School Breakfast and Lunch Programs, which serve more than 30 million students daily (USDA, 2018c).

ED plays an important role in health literacy by collecting and reporting data on health literacy, which has been associated with health outcomes (poor health literacy generally being associated with worse outcomes). According to an ED-commissioned analysis, only 12 percent of adults have a functional level of health literacy (Kutner et al., 2006)—a concern both for individuals wishing to understand the nutrition or treatment options that best meet their needs and for policy makers choosing among several health policy options. The lack of basic health literacy could overwhelm cancer patients needing to absorb an abundance of complex information throughout their care. Schools may offer partial support to alleviate this concern (which has been, as noted earlier, recognized by the United Nations Development Programme). In the United States, nearly 57 million young people are enrolled in elementary and secondary schools each year (NCES, 2018). Schools in many states already have standards in place for health education to help students learn skills to make healthful choices throughout their lifetimes, but making informed decisions during cancer treatments still remains a complex process for patients and their families.

Within the Department of the Treasury, the Alcohol and Tobacco Tax and Trade Bureau regulates the production, importation, distribution, labeling, and advertising of tobacco and alcohol—both of which are known risk factors for several malignancies. To limit the consumption of these significant cancer risk factors, the agency levies and collects excise taxes on them; however, the full effects of these tax policies on tobacco and alcohol use across the United States remain to be well characterized. Since the annual tax revenues from tobacco have been decreasing—in 2010 it was $17 billion, while in 2017 it was $14 billion—this would seem to indicate that there has been a general decline in cigarette smoking (Statista, 2018b). By comparison, revenues from alcohol sales and consumption increased over the same time, from $9.2 billion in 2010 to nearly $10 billion in 2017 (Statista, 2018a).

DOL manages workforce concerns related to employee rights and safety and also administers compensation programs for government employees—for example, DOE workers—whose work exposes them to radiation. The Bureau of Labor Statistics (BLS) publishes and maintains labor market trends. The agency has projected that the supply of physicians and surgeons will grow by 13 percent from 2016 to 2026, which is much faster than the average for all occupations. The demand for more clinicians has been expected to increase, given the aging population (BLS, 2017), but one particular analysis predicted the demand for oncology services to grow by 40 percent, whereas supply of clinicians may only grow by 25 percent through 2025 (Yang et al., 2014).

HUD's principal involvement in cancer control has been to address a wide range of environmental health and safety concerns (HUD, 2009).

The agency has implemented smoke-free policies in all its properties. In 2018, HUD expanded its mandatory no-smoking policy to all public housing and work facilities, banning the use of tobacco products in not only individual units but also common areas.

While the DOC's responsibilities are broad—it oversees international trade agreements and sets technology standards, for example—of particular relevance to cancer control is the role of its U.S. Patent and Trademark Office (USPTO). In 2016, USPTO launched the Patents 4 Patients initiative (also known as the Cancer Immunotherapy Pilot Program) to provide an accelerated review of patent applications for cancer immunotherapy technologies without a petition fee (USPTO, 2018). Between 2007 and 2017, nearly 5,400 patents were issued for cancer applications.[4] However, the bulk of these new patents have been criticized as business tactics for maintaining product market exclusivity, with claims that offer only marginal improvements and modest—or even decreased—clinical benefits to the patients who receive those drugs (Chen and Kesselheim, 2017; Hitchings et al., 2012).[5]

OMB assists the White House in setting funding priorities and in financial management across the executive branch (OMB, 2019). This broad responsibility deserves particular mention, as the OMB decisions could influence the variety and degree of cancer control activities pursued by many federal agencies. For example, since 2013, OMB's 2 percent budget sequester cut to Medicare Part B affected cancer drug reimbursement (Rosso and Davis, 2018).[6]

EEOC enforces federal laws that prohibit discrimination and harassment in the workplace. The agency enforces laws that make it illegal for private companies and federal, state, and local governments to deny a qualified job applicant a position because of a disability. Cancer patients and cancer survivors are more likely to report disputes related to job termination, terms and conditions of employment, and benefits than individuals without cancer (McKeanna et al., 2007). EEOC issues guidance on the workplace rights requiring employers to provide "reasonable accommodations" for individuals who are undergoing cancer treatments

---

[4] Results of a search in the U.S. Patent and Trademark Database with the search strategy "TTL/cancer AND ISD/20070101->20173112," from 2007 to 2017.

[5] Patents have also been sensed as a pivotal force and interact with health insurance in increasing costs of the drugs by evaporating the normal market forces. In addition, many drug patent holders employ a number of strategies, including "evergreening" and "pay for delay," to lengthen market exclusivity for their products, a topic discussed in *Making Medicines Affordable: A National Imperative* (NASEM, 2018).

[6] Several professional organizations, including the Community Oncology Alliance, have consistently filed lawsuits intended to stop CMS from applying the sequester cut because of the potential it has to shift care from community setting to outpatient hospital systems.

or have survived cancer. Such accommodations include modified work schedules or spaces for employees with cancer.

SSA offers financial support programs for thousands of cancer patients who apply for disability benefits every year. Currently, an approval of cancer-related disability claims entails a multistep process determined by the agency, based on medical reports regarding the severity of the condition and functional assessments (SSA, 2018).

OPM has the responsibility to support employee wellness, manage leave provisions, and minimize overall medical costs for the U.S. government (OPM, 2018a), which is the largest employer in the United States and spends more than $53 billion per year in medical benefits for employees and retirees (OPM, 2017). Through the Federal Employees Health Benefits Program, OPM's preventive health services coverage includes screening for breast, prostate, cervical, and colorectal cancers. The agency also provides sick leave for federal employees and their family members for conditions that require hospitalization, inpatient care, or continuing treatment. OPM's work site wellness programs and other initiatives across most federal agencies include help with smoking cessation, alcohol control, diet, and nutrition (OPM, 2018b).

From this sampling, it is clear that most of the leading agencies in the U.S. federal government—and not just those with a traditional focus on health research, wellness promotion, and disease control—are involved in cancer control efforts. And because cancer control is a complex adaptive system, the effects of these individual agencies spread widely beyond their nominal areas of responsibility.

STATE AND LOCAL INITIATIVES

The U.S. federal government has directly relied on states to design and conduct field programs for cancer control. For nearly a century, states have been recognized as principal actors for implementing a number of federal acts and initiatives on cancer, although generally without clear specifications or an overarching charter to consolidate their efforts. The National Cancer Act of 1937 required the newly formed NCI to "cooperate with state health agencies in the prevention, control, and eradication of cancer" (NCI, 2018a). The National Cancer Act of 1971 also empowered states to establish cancer control programs in collaboration with NCI (NCI, 2018b). State and territorial health departments are also periodically consulted in the formulation of the objectives for the Healthy People Initiative, a decadal priority-setting exercise for disease prevention and control. (The cancer-related goals for 2020 are listed in Box 2-1.)

Over time, as the number of participants and communities involved in cancer control efforts kept increasing, it became clear that it was not

BOX 2-1
Healthy People 2020 Objectives for Cancers

- Reduce the overall cancer death rate and death rates of lung cancer, breast cancer, cervical cancer, colorectal cancer, oropharyngeal cancer, prostate cancer, and melanoma cancer.
- Increase the number of central, population-based registries from the 50 states and the District of Columbia that capture case information on at least 95 percent of the expected number of reportable cancers.
- Increase the proportion of cancer survivors who are living 5 years or longer after diagnosis.
- Increase the mental and physical health–related quality of life of cancer survivors.
- Increase the proportion of women who receive a breast screening and cervical cancer screening or were counseled by their clinicians based on the most recent guidelines.
- Increase the proportion of men who have discussed the advantages and disadvantages of the prostate-specific antigen test to screen for prostate cancer with their clinician.
- Increase the proportion of persons who participate in behaviors that reduce their exposure to harmful ultraviolet (UV) irradiation and avoid sunburn.
- Reduce the proportion of adolescents in grades 9 through 12 who report sunburn.
- Reduce the proportion of adults aged 18 years and older who report sunburn.
- Reduce the proportion of adolescents and adults in grades 9 through 12 who report using artificial sources of UV light for tanning and increase the number of those who follow protective measures that may reduce the risk of skin cancer.

SOURCE: HHS, 2019.

enough simply to set national goals and leave it up to the multiple interested parties to determine on their own what they would do in pursuit of these goals—or even if they would pursue those goals at all. In 1998, CDC began a pilot program to promote a more "comprehensive" approach to cancer control across state, territory, and tribal administrations. In that program, CDC funded five states (Colorado, Massachusetts, Michigan, North Carolina, and Texas) and one tribal health board (Northwest Portland Area Indian Health Board), each of which already had established a cancer control plan for its jurisdiction (Major and Stewart, 2009). Cancer plans have since proliferated, and today all 50 states and the District of Columbia, 6 U.S. Pacific Island jurisdictions and Puerto Rico, and 8 tribes and tribal organizations have cancer plans in place—in total, 66.[7] Each

[7] This text has been revised since prepublication release.

plan has a local focus with whatever differences are necessary to meet local needs created by cancer burden (CDC, 2019). What is unknown is how many more unwritten, unpublished, and informal plans or guidance documents exist.[8]

CDC has determined that these plans should focus on encouraging people to make healthy choices, educating people about cancer screening tests, increasing access to high-quality cancer care, and reducing health disparities. Additionally, CDC guidance encourages plans to improve quality of life for cancer survivors, to implement changes in policies and local environments in order to promote healthy behavior, and to demonstrate outcomes through performance evaluation. It is difficult to determine whether every state pursues exactly these priorities because each state has different areas of focus, different implementation methods, different performance evaluations of their programs, and different approaches to refining and updating their plans.

Additionally, the states seem to differ on what they actually recognize as being part of the cancer control "continuum." For Arizona, the continuum includes prevention, early detection, diagnosis and treatment, quality of life, and cancer research. Alaska includes "health promotion and advocacy" and "system-level evaluation and surveillance efforts" in addition to prevention, screening and early detection, diagnosis, treatment, and survivorship. Georgia emphasizes "palliative care as needed for those living with a cancer diagnosis" along with prevention, screening and early detection, diagnosis and treatment, and survivorship.

The levels of detail in the various state cancer plans are also highly variable. In addition to high-level goals and strategies, Florida's plan also includes a variety of data sources to clarify cancer burden and apply interventions demonstrated to be useful; it also provides information on some national cancer screening guidelines. Hawaii's plan does not have explicit cancer control goals for exercise or nutrition, although these goals do appear in a companion plan focused solely on achieving them. Many state plans have a 5-year time horizon and may call for a "review" at the end of that period. The District of Columbia plan has some form of annual reviews built in over the course of its 5-year duration to aid in refining the plan as time goes on.

---

[8] For the sake of comparison, there is one national plan for cardiovascular disease, which is the number one cause of death in the United States. In 1998, Congress charged CDC to develop a national plan for heart disease and stroke and to promote the implementation of the plan in every state and U.S. territory. With the current iteration of the plan, CDC aims to help promote the achievement of national goals for preventing heart disease and stroke through 2020 and beyond.

A desired standard for a cancer control plan—or any strategic plan for health or business, for that matter—is that the goals be specific, measurable, achievable, relevant, and time bound. Some states, however, do not develop such goals for their cancer control programs, and even when such goals have been set, they are often idiosyncratic and specific to a particular state. Therefore, it is difficult if not impossible to compare goals across states and to see what kind of accountable progress is being reported from different parts of the country. A content review of the state cancer control plans revealed that Michigan, New York, and Montana, among a dozen other states, use the baseline numbers from their states' Behavioral Risk Factor Survey System (BRFSS) and Youth Risk Behavior Surveillance System (YRBSS) to set their goals and targets. For instance, to further reduce the use of tobacco products, Michigan's recently set goal is to reduce the use of smokeless tobacco products by adults and adolescents from 11.8 percent (adults) and 6.9 percent (adolescents)—the baseline values reported in the Michigan BRFSS and the YRBSS—to 10.6 percent (adults) and 6.2 percent (adolescents) by 2020. In New York, the goal is to decrease the percentage of adolescents in grades 9–12 who use any tobacco product, including e-cigarettes, from 25.4 percent—the baseline reported in the 2016 New York State Youth Tobacco Survey—to 17.7 percent by 2023. Maryland's targets are based on information from the Healthy People Initiative along with the Maryland BRFSS and the Youth Tobacco and Risk Behavior Survey.

PERFORMANCE EVALUATION

A foundational hurdle affecting the progress of state and local cancer control programs is that currently there are no agreed-upon or declared national[9] standards or methods (including for data analyses) for evaluating the performance of their cancer control plans. Each state agency, along with its coalitions or partners, is responsible for monitoring and updating its particular plan, often using standards that may be implicit or ad hoc. Furthermore, the revisions or updates—which may happen every 5 or so years, depending on the state—are generally based on some form of survey input from a wide range of participants in the state, and outside consultants may be hired to help revise and update the plans (Hager et al., 2010).

Two main techniques have been used to measure progress. In the first, the state cancer registries are consulted for data on the most recent patterns of cancer incidence, treatment, and mortality. In the second,

[9] This text has been revised since prepublication release.

data from the BRFSS,[10] the YRBSS,[11] National Immunization Surveys,[12] or the National Health and Nutrition Examination Survey (NHANES)[13] are consulted for patterns of health related behaviors that increase one's risk of cancer.[14]

Since the launch of its National Comprehensive Cancer Control Program, CDC has worked toward developing performance measures for state and local cancer plans and identifying areas of achievement as well as areas where assistance is needed (Rochester et al., 2011; Townsend et al., 2015). To develop consistent performance measurement methods, CDC established an advisory group of stakeholders and commissioned a consulting firm to prepare and implement a "logic model" that outlined structure, process, and outcome domains that might be useful for performance measures. The final worksheet produced nearly a dozen measures grouped under four main areas: engagement of stakeholder organizations, programmatic elements, funding levels, and policy outcomes. The measures have been refined over the years to clarify survey questions and strengthen indicators to more accurately measure program activities and outcomes (Townsend et al., 2015). The measures provide information about the components of the plans and their activities, the composition of the cancer control coalitions and their satisfaction, the number of objectives of the plans, and the source of their surveillance data. However, they are not able to provide meaningful information about which of the activities may not be effective and for what reasons.

The state plans have experienced mixed results, but some beneficial outcomes have been documented, including increased screening and vaccination rates and better identification of cancer survivor needs (Given et al., 2010, 2018; Rochester et al., 2010). To date, no professional organization has conducted or commissioned an objective, neutral performance analysis of all the goals proposed and implemented by state cancer control plans. On its own or under congressional directives, the Government Accountability Office (GAO) has examined the

---

[10] The BRFSS is a state-based system of telephone health surveys that collects information monthly about U.S. residents regarding their health-related risk behaviors, use of preventive health practices, and health care access related to their chronic health conditions.

[11] The YRBSS includes national, state, and local surveys conducted every 2 years to monitor the health risk behaviors among students in grades 9–12 that contribute to morbidity and mortality in both adolescence and adulthood.

[12] These surveys are a group of phone surveys used to monitor vaccination coverage among children 19–35 months and teens 13–17 years and flu vaccinations for children 6 months–17 years.

[13] NHANES includes a series of cross-sectional nationally representative health examination surveys conducted in mobile examination units or clinics to assess the health and nutritional status of children and adults in the United States.

[14] This text has been revised since prepublication release.

performance of federal health programs with particular relevance to cancer control efforts (see Box 2-2), and various changes were made in response to the GAO findings.

A VIGOROUS SYSTEM OF PARTICIPANTS AND INTERESTS

Complementing governmental efforts are hundreds of groups with diverse missions and interests, which have vigorously expanded activities for cancer control. Biopharmaceutical and medical device industries, philanthropic groups and foundations, professional organizations, academia and research organizations, employers, and, more recently, information, consumer, and financial technology companies all bring their niche, interests, and resources to this vibrant system of participants.

Currently, all large biopharmaceutical companies manufacture oncology products. Investment in cancer drug research and development has been growing strongly, forecasted to reach $100 billion by 2022 (IQVIA, 2018). Nearly 700 organizations—ranging from academic incubators and small biopharmaceutical companies with a single drug candidate to large companies with a bigger portfolio of drug candidates—have one or more oncology drugs in late-stage development (IQVIA, 2018). Oncology drugs currently represent 40 percent of the global therapeutic pipeline (Albrecht et al., 2018). And cancer products continue to dominate clinical trials—in 2017 one in every four completed industry-sponsored clinical trials was in oncology (Albrecht et al., 2018).

Funding from philanthropies and foundations for cancer control activities has also increased. One of the oldest cancer philanthropic organizations, the American Cancer Society (ACS)—created in 1945 as a successor to the American Society for the Control of Cancer—has strategically employed public relations, fund-raising, and other dynamic strategies to create a greater public demand for action on cancer. Indeed, the notion of cancer control as a "moon shot," a "winnable war," or a "crusade" was largely framed through the persistent advocacy of ACS.

Currently, nearly half of registered charities and nonprofit organizations involved in disease research, management, or advocacy in the United States are cancer related (GuideStar, 2019). These organizations generally have very narrow interests—a particular organ or tissue, a particular type of cancer, or some specific aspects of cancer control. There are multiple nonprofits focused on breast cancer, prostate cancer, lung cancer, and hospice care. Not all these "cancer" organizations have a background in medicine or population health, nor do they approach cancer control efforts through those lenses; many of them focus on socioeconomic and social justice issues or on political activism, while others are

BOX 2-2
GAO Review of Some Cancer Control Efforts

In 1980 the Government Accountability Office (GAO) conducted an analysis to determine whether the National Cancer Control Program was meeting its objectives (GAO, 1980). After reviewing some National Cancer Institute (NCI) contracts, GAO found that "NCI practices were unsound in awarding some cancer control contracts" and the contracts were not "effectively managed" and not awarded with the Department of Health, Education, and Welfare (now the Department of Health and Human Services [HHS]) procedures (GAO, 1980). In addition, the report noted that NCI was not aware of the extent that demonstration projects were continued or of the lack of cooperation between the project and contracting officers.

In 2009, GAO published its analysis of performance of the National Breast and Cervical Cancer Early Detection Program[a] and the state-level efforts to implement provisions of the Breast and Cervical Cancer Prevention and Treatment Act of 2000[b] (GAO, 2009). GAO found that only about 15 percent of eligible women in the United States received breast cancer screening through the program in 2005 and 2006. Nine percent of eligible women in the United States received cervical cancer screening from 2004 to 2006. States with more restrictive eligibility policies for the program could have had substantially fewer women screened for breast and cervical cancers. The report also found that it was difficult for women to receive financial assistance and Medicaid coverage if they received screening and diagnostic services outside the program.

More recently, GAO has continued its assessment of various public programs that have relevance to cancer control. In a 2015 report, GAO offered its analyses of 2008 and 2012 data comparing spending on cancer drugs covered under Medicare Part B at hospitals that qualified to participate in the 340B discount program to hospitals that did not qualify (GAO, 2015a). Part B spending

purely focused on the financial aspects of cancer control. Box 2-3 briefly reviews some of the roles the numerous patient advocacy groups play.

Additionally, religious institutions and faith-based organizations have played a variety of roles in cancer control (Campbell et al., 2007). Places of worship have long provided social network support to cancer patients within their congregations, chiefly through prayers, scriptural readings, and spiritual support. Many religious organizations regularly organize free cancer screening and cancer awareness programs (DeHaven et al., 2004).

Employers are paying greater attention to cancer control as they look for ways to improve the health of their employees while managing their contributions to costs for cancer care and other diseases (BLS, 2018; Isehunwa et al., 2017; Mattke et al., 2013). Box 2-4 briefly explores this topic.

on those drugs was found to be substantially higher at 340B hospitals than at non-340B hospitals.

A 2015 report from GAO estimated that the Centers for Medicare & Medicaid Services (CMS) could have substantial savings annually if the way in which Medicare pays certain cancer hospitals were modified. In a GAO comparison study, CMS was found to pay 42.3 percent more on the average for inpatient services and 37 percent more for outpatient services at 11 "comprehensive cancer centers" (as designated by NCI) than at other teaching hospitals that treat cancer with the same level of clinical complexity in the same geographic area (GAO, 2015b).

In another report issued in 2016, GAO examined HHS activities related to the Education and Awareness Requires Learning Young Act of 2014, which mandates HHS to develop and implement a national breast cancer education campaign and to support breast cancer awareness programs specifically for young women (GAO, 2016). The report found that HHS's breast cancer education campaign targeted young women. Additionally, GAO concluded that the activities employed by HHS leveraged existing resources and did not duplicate other federal breast cancer education efforts.

---

[a] The National Breast and Cervical Cancer Early Detection Program was authorized by the passage of the Breast and Cervical Cancer Mortality Prevention Act of 1990. The act authorized CDC to support states with grants to provide quality and timely breast and cervical cancer screening and diagnostic services to low-income women. The act also required CDC to provide activities including education and training for health professionals, ensuring quality of screening, and to provide evaluations of the activities. In 2000, Congress passed the Breast and Cervical Cancer Prevention and Treatment Act, which allowed states to offer women who are diagnosed with cancer through the program access to treatment through Medicaid. This footnote text has been revised since prepublication release.

[b] The act gives states the option to provide medical assistance through Medicaid to eligible women who were screened for and found to have breast or cervical cancer.

There are dozens of cancer-related professional and membership groups as well. One estimate offers a listing of nearly 58 such professional societies (CancerIndex, 2017). These various organizations frequently publish clinical practice guidelines and policy priorities for cancer control. These guidelines, as discussed in Box 2-5, often apply varying standards for evidence generation and use and sometimes make conflicting recommendations.

CONSUMER AND OTHER TECHNOLOGY FIRMS IN CANCER CONTROL

A rapidly evolving change in the U.S. health and medical system relates to the increasing direct investments and acquisitions of information, consumer, and financial technology firms by other, generally larger

BOX 2-3
Advocacy and Activism in Cancer Control

Over the decades, patient advocacy groups have very effectively brought to public awareness many diseases and their social consequences (Dresser, 2001). Besides educational activities, the various groups have particularly aided in the recruitment and participation of patients in cancer trials and have advocated for government-funded insurance and support services for cancer patients and survivors (Merkel et al., 2016). The number of such organizations advocating in the realm of cancer control far exceeds the number of groups dedicated to neurologic, cardiovascular, metabolic, and eye diseases combined (McCoy et al., 2017).

Despite their achievements, two principal concerns have been raised regarding these groups. First, the sources of funding for many of these groups are neither transparent nor readily available (Ball et al., 2006; DeJong et al., 2016; IOM, 2009; Rose, 2013). Nearly 80 percent of patient advocacy groups receive significant funding for their activities from biopharmaceutical and other technology companies, creating potential conflicts of interest (McCoy et al., 2017; Rose et al., 2017). In 2015, 14 large biopharmaceutical companies were reported to have given at least $116 million to patient advocacy groups—more than the amount the companies collectively spent on lobbying activities (Kopp et al., 2018). From these 14 companies, 6 contributed millions to individual groups that represent patients who rely on the medications produced by the companies. A recent National Academies report on the affordability of prescription drugs recommended that the Department of the Treasury should revise the Form 990 and expand the disclosure requirements on all sources of income by patient advocacy and other organizations that are exempt from income tax under the Internal Revenue Code (NASEM, 2018).

The second concern is that, in the name of activism and public awareness, organizations might aid in the diffusion of interventions before they have been shown to be more effective than current approaches, possibly also influencing the development of clinical care guidelines (Rose, 2013) (the subject of Box 2-5).

companies. Alphabet, Amazon, Apple, Facebook, GE, Google, IBM, Intel, and Microsoft are among the large companies that have active investments in health care projects, viewing this area as the next big "information business." A 2016 news report conservatively estimated that at least $40 billion in collective investment had been made by a handful of these companies (Schwartz, 2016). Coalitions have begun to emerge among wealthy donors, finance firms, and publicly traded companies, such as a recently formed entity involving Amazon, Berkshire Hathaway, and JPMorgan Chase. Google has been investing in drug development start-ups (*Reuters*, 2018), Intel has invested in predictive analytics companies working on noninvasive colon cancer screening (CB Insights, 2018), and

BOX 2-4
Workplace Wellness Programs

Employer-provided wellness programs have been seen as a way to improve employee health and to manage medical costs by preventing and reducing the burden of chronic diseases, including cancer (BLS, 2018; Isehunwa et al., 2017; Mattke et al., 2013). The Centers for Disease Control and Prevention has defined a workplace health or wellness program as "a coordinated and comprehensive set of strategies which include programs, policies, benefits, environmental supports, and links to the surrounding community designed to meet the health and safety needs of all employees" (CDC, 2018b). These employer wellness programs vary significantly in quality and purpose as well as in the health concerns they seek to address and the services they provide. A 2017 survey found that of the employers offering health benefits, 85 percent of large firms (200 or more workers) and 58 percent of small firms (3–199 workers) offered smoking cessation, alcohol control, weight management, or behavioral or lifestyle coaching wellness programs (KFF and HRET, 2017). The firms offered financial rewards such as cash, contributions to health-related savings accounts, or lowering insurance premiums as incentives for employers to participate in or complete the program.

Onsite health clinics are another tool created by employers to support employees while also controlling the expenditures associated with medical care for their employees' chronic diseases, including cancer. Known by a variety of names, such as workplace onsite health clinics or employer-based clinics, this type of employer service is not new. Such services have existed since the 1930s at coal mines, construction sites, and steel mills, for instance (Stephens, 2018). A 2015 survey of 120 U.S.-based companies offering or planning to offer onsite health clinics reported that 86 percent offered new services that included lifestyle and wellness programs, while nearly all offered immunizations and acute care services (Towers Watson, 2015). Nearly half the centers offered pharmacy services, while 35 percent offered virtual medical consultation. Almost all the respondents noted convenience for employees and a decrease in time away from work as major objectives met.

Microsoft is investing in improved cancer diagnostics (Microsoft News Center India, 2018). Many of these companies also bring to bear significantly advanced computational capabilities previously unavailable for any application in society.

In the next decade or so, if forecasts are correct, the already complex cancer control system will gain an entire new layer of complexity with the large-scale aggregation of genomic, environmental, behavioral, and other information from representative patient populations. The purpose of collecting these vast amounts of diverse data is to enable the creation of treatments tailored to the unique biology of individual patients. Underlying these initiatives are new computational capabilities for rapidly conducting

BOX 2-5
Variations in Clinical Practice Guidelines

One of the clearest indications of the complexity of—and lack of integration in—today's cancer care system is the variation in clinical practice guidelines. From the patient's point of view, it would be preferable to have one agreed-upon answer to such questions as "How often should I be screened for breast cancer?" or "Should I get tested for prostate cancer?" But currently there is no such agreement, and that can lead to confusion and uneven delivery of cancer care.

Consider breast cancer screening. In 2016, the U.S. Preventive Services Task Force (USPSTF) recommended that women aged 50–74 with "average risk" for breast cancer undergo screening mammography every 2 years (Siu, 2016). In contrast, the 2017 American College of Obstetricians and Gynecologists guideline recommends screening of average risk women beginning at age 40 through age 75 and leaves the interval of screening (annually or biennially) to be determined by the patients in discussion with their clinicians (Mango et al., 2018). Similarly, the American Cancer Society (ACS) calls for screening to be initiated at age 45 and done yearly through age 54 and biennially after that. The ACS guideline also states that women aged 40–44 should have the choice to begin annual screening. It does not recommend a firm upper limit in age beyond which screening is not advised but rather recommends screening cessation when life expectancy is less than 10 years (Smith et al., 2018). The National Comprehensive Cancer Network (NCCN), the American College of Radiology, and the Society of Breast Imaging also recommend annual mammography starting at age 40 but differ in their recommendations concerning screening cessation. Specifically, the American College of Radiology does not recommend mammography when the patient's life expectancy is less than 10 years, whereas the Society of Breast Imaging does not recommend mammography when the patient's life expectance is less than 5–7 years (Mango et al., 2018). Thus, five different guidelines for mammography have been issued by five different authorities on women's health or cancer care.

The differences arise because of differences in how the various organizations weigh the potential benefits of screening versus the potential harms, such as unnecessary biopsies and treatments, but it can be very difficult for patients to see the disagreements as anything less than contradictory and confusing. A similar situation exists with the guidelines for prostate cancer screening. In 2012, the USPSTF recommended against prostate-specific antigen (PSA)-based screening in men of any age (Moyer, 2012). The rationale was that published data do not support the hypothesis that most asymptomatic prostate cancer cases will become clinically important or that early treatment, which is associated with significant morbidity, reduces the prostate cancer–specific health burden or mortality from prostate cancer. In contrast, the following year, the American Urological Association concluded that the harms of PSA testing were outweighed by potential benefits for patients aged 55–69 years and recommended "shared decision making" with clinicians based on the men's values and preferences (American Urological Association, 2018). The American College of Physicians issued a similar recommendation (Qaseem et al., 2013), while ACS recommended PSA screening starting at age 50, not 55 (Smith et al., 2018). The European Association of Urology went on to recommend baseline PSA measurement starting at age 40 (Heidenreich et al., 2013).

The controversy prompted an international convention in Australia to address the confusion over PSA testing, resulting in the Melbourne Consensus Statement. This statement recommended baseline PSA measurement for men in their 40s and stated that PSA testing does reduce the incidence of metastatic prostate cancer as well as prostate cancer–specific mortality rates for men aged 50–69 (Murphy et al., 2014). To temper its refutation of the USPSTF recommendation, the Melbourne statement did recommend that prostate cancer diagnosis be uncoupled from prostate cancer intervention, a nod to the growing data to support the use of active surveillance rather than treatment for low-risk prostate cancer (Loeb, 2014). Most recently, the USPSTF recommended that for men aged 55–69, the decision to have PSA screening should be an "individual one" based on discussion with their clinician about the potential benefits and harms in relationship to their own preferences and values; for men age 70 and over, the task force continues to advise against PSA screening (USPSTF, 2018).

There are also variations in the guidelines for the diagnostic workup and treatment of cancer. Even within a single guideline resource, such as NCCN, many clinical situations have more than one option from which patients and clinicians can choose (NCCN, 2018). Many societies and guideline-issuing organizations advocate for "shared decision making" between patients and clinicians to arrive at cancer care decisions when there is more than one option, giving patients the deciding vote. However, the reliance on "shared decision making," while seemingly a positive for the patient, can open the door to powerful and perverse financial incentives that can subtly influence the recommendations that clinicians give patients.

The conundrum is as follows: fewer screening tests means fewer laboratory tests, fewer diagnostic radiology studies, and fewer biopsies. While individual clinicians, in general, are intrinsically motivated toward what is best for their patients, oncology practices are rapidly transitioning from clinician-owned practices toward health system–owned practices (Clough et al., 2017). Thus, clinicians often have volume-based performance benchmarks set by their employers seeking to measure productivity. Benchmarks may consist of quantity-of-care metrics such as the number of cases operated, the number of films read, and the number of work relative value units, with the bottom line being that more interventions are associated with better performance. This creates a scenario in which busy clinicians are dedicating themselves to often time-consuming discussions with patients to make shared decisions about care while also needing to meet the benchmarks by which their performance is judged or compensation, directly or indirectly, is derived.

Another source of confusion for patients arises from "medical reversals," when clinical guidelines are suddenly changed based on new information. These are common in medical practice and contribute to inconsistent advice given by clinicians, widespread variation in practice patterns that is not justified by evidence, and potential harm to patients (Prasad, 2016).

whole-genome sequencing, identifying novel associations (e.g., through machine learning), and linking these associations to patient outcomes. With large patient databases, it is also possible to understand whether unusual treatment responses identified in small patient populations point toward previously unrecognized patient populations who could benefit from tailored treatments (Chakradhar, 2016).

In the past decade, several major public and private ventures have been launched with the goal of creating repositories of genomic data that can be sequenced and analyzed. The NIH Cancer Genome Atlas, launched in 2006, has the goal to "generate, quality control, merge, analyze, and interpret molecular profiles at the DNA, RNA, protein, and epigenetic levels for hundreds of clinical tumors representing various tumor types and their subtypes" (Weinstein et al., 2013). By the end of the program in 2018, the Cancer Genome Atlas had mapped nearly 20,000 specimens spanning 33 cancer types (NCI, 2019). The Cancer Genome Atlas Research Network has provided the infrastructure (through joint funding by NIH and European agencies) to archive these data (Tomczak et al., 2015). Along with NIH's All of Us program, VA's Million Veteran Program, and nongovernmental programs such as the Oncology Research Information Exchange Network, there seem to be numerous promising opportunities to harness computation tools to advance cancer control. Google's Verily, for example, has already demonstrated a proof of concept for using "deep learning" approaches to identify the location and size of a breast cancer tumor in a way that can outperform human radiologists (Dobush, 2018).

The inevitable rise of such large-scale data approaches to cancer research will require further efforts to develop aggregation infrastructure to share these insights widely. However, these data collection and storage mechanisms have begun to raise a host of questions related to equity (e.g., Who benefits from the new knowledge?), access (e.g., Do patients have the right to refuse the uses and reuses of their data?), and commercialization (e.g., Do all uses of data need to have an altruistic objective, or can these data be used for private, commercial benefit?).

HISTORICALLY COMMON THEMES

Several themes have commonly appeared and been regularly repeated in discussions on cancer control over the past couple of decades. Drawing on previous publications of the National Academies, six of those common themes are summarized in this section.

The first theme is the very "fragmented" nature of cancer control efforts—one that affects patients in significant ways and makes it logistically challenging to coordinate actions across the cancer control continuum, including prevention, screening and early detection, diagnosis, treatment, palliative care, survivorship care, and hospice care (IOM, 2001a, 2003a,b, 2006, 2007, 2008, 2013a,b, 2015). The usual recommendations to address this fragmentation have been to encourage better integration and coordination among cancer programs, hospital and social services, and clinicians and to provide more funding from government and private agencies to drive that coordination. Two reports, for example, made identical recommendations that funding agencies should support work to enable continuous coordination between cancer treatment and survivorship care (IOM, 2003b, 2006). Other recommendations have called for consistency among clinical practice guidelines and assessment tools.

The second theme is improving cancer prevention and early detection. Recommendations have included expanding screening programs, increasing vaccination rates, and promoting public awareness and education (IOM, 2001a, 2003a, 2007; NASEM, 2016a). Insurance companies have been encouraged to provide coverage for cancer prevention and early detection (IOM, 2003c), and federal and state agencies have been urged to expand community-based programs that provide hepatitis B screening, testing, and vaccination services (IOM, 2010b). There have also been regular calls for increased public–private partnerships to promote healthy lifestyles.

The third theme is the availability and use of a "data infrastructure"—an issue that routinely comes up not only in discussions on how to understand and improve cancer control efforts but also in more general discussions about overall medical care and health policy. "There is no national cancer care data system in the United States," concluded an Institute of Medicine report issued in 2000 (IOM, 2000a). Today, there is still no such system. Frequently cited reasons for the lack of such a data system include the absence of recognized quality measures, the absence of benchmarks to measure progress, and concerns about the confidentiality and security of patient information. Various recommendations have called for improving regulations governing the collection and use of clinical patient data (IOM, 1999, 2000a, 2014), while another typical recommendation has called for the development of "patient portals" to enhance data sharing and communication among clinicians, patients, and families (IOM, 2013a). The development of a data infrastructure that is widely available can be seen as a separate approach to increasing coordination—another goal that appears repeatedly in various forms.

A fourth theme concerns the persistent health disparities that exist in cancer control. Specific recommendations have been to identify and disseminate effective community interventions, to support public–private initiatives to reduce disparities in the cancer burden, and to develop specific programs and initiatives to increase access to medical services (IOM, 1999, 2013b). There have also been calls to ensure consistent implementation of current standards of care and measurement of quality metrics (IOM, 2003b, 2013b; NASEM, 2016a).

A fifth theme is the importance of biomarkers and new technologies for chemoprevention, early detection, disease classification, drug development, treatment planning, and monitoring and surveillance (IOM, 2001b, 2003a, 2007, 2010a). Biomarkers are essential for the success of precision medicine approaches to cancer treatment (NASEM, 2016b), which aim to improve the safety and effectiveness of interventions by increasing response rates, reducing adverse effects of therapy, and increasing patient adherence to treatment regimens (Burnette et al., 2012; Collins and Varmus, 2015; Love-Koh et al., 2018; Savoia et al., 2017; Snyderman, 2014). However, precision medicine has also been met with some skepticism about whether its potential to improve patient outcomes can be fully achieved. A 2016 National Academies report on biomarker tests for precision medicine emphasized the importance of standards for evidence generation, oversight, payment models, and decision making for test development and use in clinical care (NASEM, 2016b).

The absence of agreement on the precise definition of precision approaches—now being extended to prevention—also poses uncertainty from a regulatory and reimbursement standpoint (Degtiar, 2017; Faulkner et al., 2012). Another challenge in achieving the goals of precision medicine is that precision approaches do not typically consider the larger social environment of the individuals—a factor that some consider to be at least as influential as genetics for the design of various treatments (Bayer and Galea, 2015; Carlsten et al., 2014; Juengst et al., 2016; Minari et al., 2018). One argument for greater investments in population health—versus precision medicine—seems to stem in part from the disparities in the occurrence and outcomes of disease as noted above, with certain groups more likely to develop the disease or less likely to receive effective treatment or both.

The sixth theme is about making cancer research and care more effective and efficient (IOM, 2000b). Recommendations have focused on improving the process of conducting large-scale biomedical research (IOM, 2003d), developing guidance on reimbursement decisions (IOM, 2006), determining the factors that put individuals at high risk for poor physical and psychosocial outcomes (IOM, 2008), identifying effective ways to communicate accurate cancer risk information and statistics to patients and other stakeholders (IOM, 2012), and enabling the broader enrollment of patients in clinical trials (IOM, 2010c). All six themes have been linked to calls for more research and more coordination.

PUBLIC TRUST IN CANCER CONTROL

New discoveries often spur changes in clinical and public health practice, drive the creation of new academic subfields, and shift funding priorities for research and product development. Some putative discoveries, however, have later been shown to be irreproducible, ultimately setting back scientific progress and delaying potential benefits for patients. A growing body of evidence indicates that study findings in the biomedical, public health, and social sciences often cannot be replicated. This is a topic of active concern in the scientific community and policy circles.

In a recent survey, greater than 70 percent of researchers reported that they had tried and failed to reproduce another researcher's experiments at some point. In addition, greater than half of the researchers had failed to reproduce some of their own experiments (Baker, 2016). This issue of reproducibility further complicates the clinical guidelines debate and raises concerns about whether the right kinds of investments are being made in research and whether research is accountable and responsive to such investments, often coming from taxpayers (An, 2018). A recent report on reproducibility and replicability in science recommended that "scientists should take care to avoid overstating the implications of their research and also exercise caution in their review of press releases, especially when the results bear directly on matters of keen public interest and possible action" and that "anyone making personal or policy decisions based on scientific evidence should be wary of making a serious decision based on the results, no matter how promising, of a single study" (NASEM, 2019).

False-positive results stem from two factors: a lack of statistical power and experimental or investigator bias. Recent analyses have shown that false-positive results are even more likely to appear in circumstances where multiple research teams are simultaneously testing the same hypothesis (e.g., in genome-wide sequencing studies), where it is likely that at least one research team will find a significant result purely by chance (Ioannidis, 2005). Compounding this challenge is the fact that the scientific community and the current academic incentives tend to reward positive findings more strongly than negative findings, which might motivate a minority of researchers to inappropriately manipulate study designs or misrepresent data in ways that increase the chances of obtaining positive results (recognized in the scientific community as misconduct, similar to data fabrication) (NASEM, 2017). Several aspects of study design can contribute to bias and false-positive results. For example, findings with small effect sizes (even when statistically significant) are more likely to be false-positive results. In addition, allowing for more flexibility in design, definition, and acceptable testing strategies can also lead to post hoc, arbitrary changes to study design that can alter results (known as "*p*-hacking") (Ioannidis, 2005). For example, some investigators might alter sample inclusion criteria after data are collected, which could increase the likelihood of finding a positive effect. In cancer prognostic studies, it was found that inconsistent reporting of patient outcomes was likely to introduce bias in study findings that could spuriously inflate the significance of prognostic factors (Kyzas et al., 2005). Bias can be inferred by the number of published studies with *p*-values that irregularly cluster around the "$p < 0.05$" value (Head et al., 2015). Many scholars have advocated for greater prespecification of study designs in both observational and controlled trials to reduce the likelihood that study design can be manipulated to achieve positive results (Head et al., 2015). Recently, more than 800 researchers from more than 50 countries also proposed abandoning the use of statistical significance to decide whether a result refutes or supports a scientific hypothesis (Amrhein et al., 2019).

Reproducibility problems arise in several subfields relating to cancer control for different reasons, perhaps notably because of the sheer biological complexity of the system under analysis. A 2012 *Nature* editorial argued that success in oncology drug development has been limited by unreliable results from preclinical studies, with reference to a report that Amgen scientists were only able to replicate 11 percent of study findings from 53 landmark studies in hematology and oncology (Begley and Ellis, 2012). This lack of study replication may be due in part to inadequate descriptions of the experimental methods and variability in techniques or cell line and mouse models, but regardless of the cause, the implications are significant. Translating preclinical findings to human trials, which often focus on survival as an end point, requires a substantial investment of resources and time. Thus, accurate and reliable preclinical results are critical for advancing progress in the field.

Challenges with the reproducibility of study findings also arise in fields that rely on the mining of large, observational data sets. For example, nutritional epidemiology studies often make the headlines for identifying associations between dietary intake and cancer risk, but the results from different studies may be contradictory. Coffee, as one example, has been reported to either increase or reduce the risks of cancers—and Parkinson's disease—depending on the study (Carroll, 2015). The results also vary depending on the populations studied, how the exposure and end points are assessed, and what statistical tools were used. A systematic review of studies that sampled 50 ingredients commonly listed in cookbooks found that 80 percent of these ingredients had been studied in relation to risk of cancer, with 39 percent of the studies reporting increased risk, 33 percent reporting decreased risk, and 23 percent showing no evidence of either increased or decreased risk (Schoenfeld and Ioannidis, 2012).

As these examples illustrate, it is difficult to document, verify, and accurately communicate information to the public and policy makers about cancer risk factors and interventions. Public confidence in and, ultimately, public support for research on cancer control—from epidemiology to economics—could be compromised by the dissemination of poor-quality evidence.

Moreover, recent media headlines highlight three new developments in cancer care and research that also have the potential to influence public trust. First is the increased and questionable promotion of services directly to patients by some medical centers and the rapidly growing marketing expenditures of drugs by biopharmaceutical companies (see Box 2-6 for additional discussion on promotion of cancer services and products). The second development is the lack of full disclosure by some researchers of financial ties to for-profit companies and other interested parties. Recent news reports have centered on medical leaders (including a chief executive officer and a chief medical officer of a renowned cancer center and a dean of a prominent medical school) who failed to disclose their financial relationships with biopharmaceutical and medical businesses in multiple publications (Ornstein and Thomas, 2018). This does not necessarily mean that the results from their published research are inaccurate, but the lack of responsible disclosure—a long-standing concern in biomedical and related research—could adversely influence public trust in cancer research. The third development is violation of anti-kickback laws by drug manufacturers, highlighted by a case in which one drug manufacturer effectively used donations and patient advocacy groups to subsidize drug costs for patients enrolled in Medicare (Thomas, 2018). Federal anti-kickback laws prohibit this practice.

TOWARD A CONSOLIDATED VISION

What can be seen from this chapter's brief overview is that the cancer control system—in the United States but also in the rest of the world—is a collection of many individual components, only minimally integrated, that has been built up over time with little overarching vision or strategy and yielding varied results. However, despite the vital importance of cancer control in terms of both its financial and social costs, no one has yet applied a systems approach to the cancer control system in any comprehensive way.

As described in the next chapter, there have been efforts to understand certain individual components of the cancer control system—tobacco control and survivorship, for instance—with systems analysis, but those cannot answer questions about the entire cancer control system. For example, there has never been a serious attempt to analyze prevention and

BOX 2-6
Promotion of Cancer Services and Products

Direct-to-consumer marketing of medical services is a multibillion-dollar industry in the United States. One analysis found that direct-to-consumer advertising spending by U.S. cancer centers increased three-fold from 2005 to 2014, and of the $173 million spent on advertising in 2014, 86 percent came from just 20 centers comprising for-profit centers and those accredited as NCI-Designated Cancer Centers (Vater et al., 2016). A recent examination of marketing materials of 50 cancer centers that spent the most on advertising in 2017 indicated that some of the promotional tactics used included conveying an unrealistic sense of hope to patients about survival chances using powerful testimonials, including paid actors (TINA, 2018). Sometimes the narratives offer an assurance to patients that treatment at a specific cancer center will provide patients with a therapeutic advantage, allowing them to beat the odds and live beyond 5 years. Some of the advertisements also promote their ongoing clinical trials as well as "novel treatments" without necessarily disclosing the associated risks.

The direct-to-consumer marketing tactic is clearly not unique to medical centers. Advertising of prescription drugs directly to consumers occupies more than half of the total direct-to-consumer expenditures for all medical services and products (Schwartz and Woloshin, 2019). Direct-to-consumer advertising of cancer drugs particularly have increased rapidly from only about $3 million in 1997 to $274 million annually. Although the expenditure on cancer drugs accounts for only a part of the trends, it nevertheless exceeds that of respiratory medications ($255 million), immunology medications ($218 million), and cholesterol medications ($48 million), and the current trends indicate that spending to advertise cancer drugs to consumers is only going to continue to increase (Schwartz and Woloshin, 2019).

As discussed in a previous National Academies report, proponents of direct-to-consumer advertising view it as a service by educating and empowering people

treatment efforts as part of the same interconnected system and to determine what combination of prevention and treatment strategies will have the greatest benefit for a given cost. Doing so will require a completely different approach to better understanding and shaping a system using the approaches and tools of systems engineering.

FINDINGS

Finding 2-1: *Historically, national strategic plans have been successfully established and refined to meet the prioritized needs of population health, national security, transportation, and economic development over the past century. However, the development of an overarching, unified national strategic vision for cancer control in the United States has been particularly impeded by the sheer* with information to make better health and medical choices, with claims that it aids proper medication use and adherence. Critics—including some who advocate to ban this practice—argue that the advertisements are of no value beyond boosting corporate revenues. The advertisements can influence patients to request prescriptions from their clinicians, which can lead to overuse of expensive products and services that may not offer any additional benefits (NASEM, 2018).

The Congressional Budget Office (CBO) has examined the anticipated effects of a moratorium on this sort of advertising (CBO, 2011):

- Drug manufacturers would probably expand their marketing to clinicians to substitute for at least some of the banned advertising to consumers.
- The number of prescriptions filled would probably decrease for some drugs, but for other drugs the number of prescriptions might be little changed, owing both to the likely substitution of other types of promotions and to other factors that influence a drug's reach in the prescription drug market.
- Any change in prescription drug prices would depend on changes in demand; however, prices for new brand drugs that normally would be part of a direct-to-consumer advertising campaign could increase, since sales would be reduced.
- A moratorium could affect public health. The exact result would depend on whether the benefits of fewer unexpected adverse health events were greater than the health costs of possibly reduced use of new and effective drugs.

The various scenarios described by CBO are exactly the sort of things one would expect from an adaptive system responding to a stimulus (elimination of direct-to-consumer advertising): drug manufacturers, consumers, and doctors would all modify their behavior in various ways to account for this change. Therefore finding a solution will require an understanding of the emerging behavior of the entire system rather than isolating and focusing on individual parts.

variety of participants and their programmatic, financial, professional, and other motivations.

Finding 2-2: *In the United States, various initiatives pertaining to cancer control involve the leadership of at least a dozen federal government agencies in addition to those principally focused on health promotion, disease control, and medical benefits.*

Finding 2-3: *Cancer control activities in the United States involve hundreds of participant groups with diverse interests. Among these, as a few examples, are biopharmaceutical firms engaged in research and product development efforts, numerous professional societies setting clinical guidelines, and nonprofit patient and research advocates and individual activists.*

Finding 2-4: *Currently, there are at least 65 known strategic plans for cancer control across states, tribes, and territories in the United States. These contextual plans lack an integrated framework, each involving different review processes, outcomes analyses, and reporting requirements.*

Finding 2-5: *Currently, each state sets its own objectives and indicates how these goals were derived. Moreover, there are no criteria for what constitutes an adequate state cancer control plan.*

Finding 2-6: *At all levels of cancer control planning in the United States, currently no widely agreed-upon systematic standards and procedures exist to enable comprehensive performance reviews of programs and interventions, interactive monitoring of trends, and joint action for contingencies.*

Finding 2-7: *The current cancer control system does not provide sufficient transparency to enable a clear understanding of the potential financial influences and conflict of interests between participants such as researchers, clinicians, drug, device, and other product manufacturers as well as patient advocates and their organizations. Although a long-recognized concern, lack of public reporting of these financial relationships could continue to compromise the integrity of efforts and affect the progress in cancer control.*

Finding 2-8: *The current trends in the production and dissemination of information through interest groups and new forms of media and social channels—including direct marketing and advertising of products and services—can lead to a profusion of conflicting and confusing messages for patients seeking pertinent information. Promotional messages using questionable tactics to hype the benefits of their products or services run the risk of misleading patients.*

Finding 2-9: *Reliable evidence is a vital prerequisite for cancer research, care, and policies and, ultimately, population health. However, it is crucial that research results and publications in biomedical, public health, social and behavioral sciences, and related areas meet the central scientific standards of reproducibility and replicability required to maintain the public confidence and support, all essential for effective cancer control.*

Finding 2-10: *Clinical guidelines currently issued by numerous advisory and professional organizations for cancer screening and care in the United States widely diverge from one another even for a specific cancer type. These inconsistencies may lead to adverse consequences for patients and increase the financial waste in care.*

REFERENCES

AHRQ (Agency for Healthcare Research and Quality). 2019. *About AHRQ.* https://www.ahrq.gov/cpi/about/index.html (accessed February 15, 2019).

Albrecht, B., S. Andersen, K. Chauhan, D. Graybosch, and P. Menu. 2018. *Pursuing breakthroughs in cancer-drug development.* https://www.mckinsey.com/industries/pharmaceuticals-and-medical-products/our-insights/pursuing-breakthroughs-in-cancer-drug-development (accessed February 15, 2019).

American Urological Association. 2018. *Early detection of prostate cancer.* https://www.auanet.org/guidelines/prostate-cancer-early-detection-guideline (accessed February 15, 2019).

Amrhein, V., S. Greenland, and B. McShane. 2019. Scientists rise up against statistical significance. *Nature* 567(7748):305.

An, G. 2018. The crisis of reproducibility, the denominator problem and the scientific role of multi-scale modeling. *Bulletin* of *Mathematical Biology* 80(12):3071–3080.

Baker, M. 2016. 1,500 scientists lift the lid on reproducibility. *Nature* 533(7604):452–454.

Ball, D. E., K. Tisocki, and A. Herxheimer. 2006. Advertising and disclosure of funding on patient organisation websites: A cross-sectional survey. *BMC Public Health* 6:201.

Bayer, R., and S. Galea. 2015. Public health in the precision-medicine era. *New England Journal of Medicine* 373(6):499–501.

Begley, C. G., and L. M. Ellis. 2012. Drug development: Raise standards for preclinical cancer research. *Nature* 483(7391):531–533.

BLS (Bureau of Labor Statistics). 2017. *Physicians and surgeons.* https://www.bls.gov/ooh/healthcare/physicians-and-surgeons.htm (accessed February 15, 2019).

BLS. 2018. *Employee access to wellness programs in 2017.* https://www.bls.gov/opub/ted/2018/employee-access-to-wellness-programs-in-2017.htm (accessed February 15, 2019).

Bray, F., J. Ferlay, I. Soerjomataram, R. L. Siegel, L. A. Torre, and A. Jemal. 2018. Global cancer statistics 2018: Globocan estimates of incidence and mortality worldwide for 36 cancers in 185 countries. *CA: A Cancer Journal for Clinicians* 68(6):394–424.

Burnette, R., L. A. Simmons, and R. Snyderman. 2012. Personalized health care as a pathway for the adoption of genomic medicine. *Journal of Personalized Medicine* 2(4):232–240.

Campbell, M. K., M. A. Hudson, K. Resnicow, N. Blakeney, A. Paxton, and M. Baskin. 2007. Church-based health promotion interventions: Evidence and lessons learned. In *Annual Review of Public Health* 28:213–234.

CancerIndex. 2017. *National organisations: USA.* http://www.cancerindex.org/clinks5n.htm (accessed February 15, 2019).

Carlsten, C., M. Brauer, F. Brinkman, J. Brook, D. Daley, K. McNagny, M. Pui, D. Royce, T. Takaro, and J. Denburg. 2014. Genes, the environment and personalized medicine: We need to harness both environmental and genetic data to maximize personal and population health. *EMBO Reports* 15(7):736–739.

Carroll, A. 2015. *More consensus on coffee's effect on health than you might think.* https://www.nytimes.com/2015/05/12/upshot/more-consensus-on-coffees-benefits-than-you-might-think.html (accessed February 15, 2019).

CB Insights. 2018. *Where big tech is placing bets in healthcare.* https://www.healthcare.digital/single-post/2017/12/28/CB-Insights-Where-Big-Tech-Is-Placing-Bets-In-Healthcare (accessed February 15, 2019).

CBO (Congressional Budget Office). 2011. *Potential effects of a ban on direct-to-consumer advertising of new prescription drugs.* May 26. Washington, DC: Congressional Budget Office. https://www.cbo.gov/publication/41449 (accessed February 15, 2019).

CBPP (Center on Budget and Policy Priorities). 2018. *A closer look at who benefits from SNAP: State-by-state fact sheets.* https://www.cbpp.org/research/food-assistance/a-closer-look-at-who-benefits-from-snap-state-by-state-fact-sheets?fa=view&id=3886#Alabama (accessed February 15, 2019).

CDC (Centers for Disease Control and Prevention). 2018a. *National programs.* https://www.cdc.gov/cancer/dcpc/about/programs.htm (accessed February 15, 2019).

CDC. 2018b. *Workplace health model.* https://www.cdc.gov/workplacehealthpromotion/model/index.html (accessed February 15, 2019).

CDC. 2019. *About the National Comprehensive Cancer Control Program.* https://www.cdc.gov/cancer/ncccp/about.htm (accessed February 15, 2019).

Census Bureau. 2018. *Veteran population.* https://www.census.gov/newsroom/facts-for-features/2018/veterans-day.html (accessed February 15, 2019).

Chakradhar, S. 2016. Group mentality: Determining if targeted treatments really work for cancer. *Nature Medicine* 22(3):222–224.

Chen, C. T., and A. S. Kesselheim. 2017. Journey of generic imatinib: A case study in oncology drug pricing: *Journal of Oncology Practice*, 13(6):352.

Clough, J. D., M. A. Dinan, and K. A. Schulman. 2017. Trends in hospital-physician integration in medical oncology. *American Journal of Managed Care* 23(10):624–627.

Cohen, P. 2015. DARPA's Big Mechanism Program. *Physical Biology* 12(4):045008.

Collins, F. S., and H. Varmus. 2015. A new initiative on precision medicine. *New England Journal of Medicine* 372(9):793–795.

Degtiar, I. 2017. A review of international coverage and pricing strategies for personalized medicine and orphan drugs. *Health Policy* 121(12):1240–1248.

DeHaven, M. J., I. B. Hunter, L. Wilder, J. W. Walton, and J. Berry. 2004. Health programs in faith-based organizations: Are they effective? *American Journal of Public Health* 94(6):1030–1036.

DeJong, C., T. Aguilar, C. W. Tseng, G. A. Lin, W. J. Boscardin, and R. A. Dudley. 2016. Pharmaceutical industry-sponsored meals and physician prescribing patterns for Medicare beneficiaries. *JAMA Internal Medicine* 176(8):1114–1122.

Dobush, G. 2018. *Google's AI tool can identify one type of breast cancer more accurately than human doctors.* http://fortune.com/2018/10/15/google-ai-metastatic-breast-cancer (accessed February 15, 2019).

DoD (Department of Defense). 2015. *Congressionally directed medical research programs.* https://cdmrp.army.mil/researchprograms (accessed February 15, 2019).

DOE (Department of Energy). 2018. *Energy Department advances supercomputing in fight against cancer.* https://www.energy.gov/articles/energy-department-advances-supercomputing-fight-against-cancer (accessed February 15, 2019).

Dresser, R. 2001. *When science offers salvation: Patient advocacy and research ethics.* New York: Oxford University Press.

Economist Intelligence Unit. 2015. *Controlling cancer: The state of national cancer control plans in Asia.* http://www.mundipharma.com.sg/wp-content/uploads/2016/02/5488e16a8d094e77a161e178f754a09e1.pdf?569680 (accessed February 15, 2019).

EPA (Environmental Protection Agency). 2018. *Laws and regulations.* https://www.epa.gov/laws-regulations (accessed February 15, 2019).

Faulkner, E., L. Annemans, L. Garrison, M. Helfand, A.-P. Holtorf, J. Hornberger, D. Hughes, T. Li, D. Malone, and K. Payne. 2012. Challenges in the development and reimbursement of personalized medicine—payer and manufacturer perspectives and implications for health economics and outcomes research: A report of the ISPOR personalized medicine special interest group. *Value in Health* 15(8):1162–1171.

FDA (Food and Drug Administration). 2018. *Oncology Center of Excellence*. https://www.fda.gov/AboutFDA/CentersOffices/OfficeofMedicalProductsandTobacco/OCE/default.htm (accessed February 15, 2019).

GAO (Government Accountability Office). 1980. *The objectives of the cancer control program and the National Cancer Institute's administration of program contracts*. HRD-80-57. June. Washington, DC: Government Accountability Office.

GAO. 2009. *Medicaid: Source of screening affects women's eligibility for coverage of breast and cervical cancer treatment in some states*. GAO-09-384. May. Washington, DC: Government Accountability Office.

GAO. 2015a. *Action needed to reduce financial incentives to prescribe 340B drugs at participating hospitals*. GAO-15-442. June. Washington, DC: Government Accountability Office.

GAO. 2015b. *Medicare: Payment methods for certain cancer hospitals should be revised to promote efficiency*. GAO-15-199. February. Washington, DC: Government Accountability Office.

GAO. 2016. *Breast cancer education: HHS has implemented initiatives aimed at young women*. GAO-17-19. October. Washington, DC: Government Accountability Office.

Given, L. S., K. Hohman, L. Graaf, P. Rochester, and L. Belle-Isle. 2010. From planning to implementation to outcomes: Comprehensive cancer control implementation building blocks. *Cancer Causes and Control* 21(12):1987–1994.

Given, L. S., R. Coughlin, P. Hager, K. Lopez, G. Merriam, K. Morwood, D. Nelson, and A. Crawford. 2018. Comprehensive cancer control in the US: 20 years of progress. *Cancer Causes and Control* 29(12):1151.

GuideStar. 2019. *Directory of charities and nonprofit organizations*. https://www.guidestar.org/search (accessed February 15, 2019).

Hager, P., L. Given, J. Redmond, and K. Rogers. 2010. Revision of comprehensive cancer control plans: Experiences shared by three states. *Cancer Causes and Control* 21(12):2005–2013.

Hanyuda, T. 2012. *Cancer control in Japan*. https://www.med.or.jp/english/journal/pdf/2012_06/501_503.pdf (accessed February 15, 2019).

Head, M. L., L. Holman, R. Lanfear, A. T. Kahn, and M. D. Jennions. 2015. The extent and consequences of *p*-hacking in science. *PLoS Biology* 13(3):e1002106.

Heidenreich, A., P. A. Abrahamsson, W. Artibani, J. Catto, F. Montorsi, H. Van Poppel, M. Wirth, and N. Mottet. 2013. Early detection of prostate cancer: European Association of Urology recommendation. *European Urology* 64(3):347–354.

HHS (Department of Health and Human Services). 2018. *Reproductive health*. https://www.hhs.gov/opa/reproductive-health/index.html (accessed February 15, 2019).

HHS. 2019. *Healthy People 2020*. https://www.healthypeople.gov/2020/topics-objectives/topic/cancer (accessed February 15, 2019).

Hitchings, A. W., E. H. Baker, and T. K. Khong. 2012. Making medicines evergreen. *British Medical Journal* 345:e7941.

HRSA (Health Resources and Services Administration). 2019. *About HRSA*. https://www.hrsa.gov/about/index.html (accessed February 15, 2019).

HUD (Department of Housing and Urban Development). 2009. *Leading our nation to healthier homes: The healthy homes strategic plan*. https://www.hud.gov/sites/dfiles/HH/documents/hh_strategic_plan.web_posting.pdf (accessed February 15, 2019).

IHS (Indian Health Service). 2019. *Health issues—cancer*. https://ihs.gov/epi/cancer (accessed February 15, 2019).

Ioannidis, J. P. 2005. Why most published research findings are false. *PLoS Medicine* 2(8):e124.

IOM (Institute of Medicine).1999. *Ensuring quality cancer care*. Washington, DC: National Academy Press.

IOM. 2000a. *Enhancing data systems to improve the quality of cancer care*. Washington, DC: National Academy Press.

IOM. 2000b. *Promoting health: Intervention strategies from social and behavioral research*. Washington, DC: National Academy Press.
IOM. 2001a. *Mammography and beyond: Developing technologies for the early detection of breast cancer*. Washington, DC: National Academy Press.
IOM. 2001b. *Improving palliative care: We can take better care of people with cancer*. Washington, DC: National Academy Press.
IOM. 2003a. *Fulfilling the potential of cancer prevention and early detection*. Washington, DC: The National Academies Press.
IOM. 2003b. *Childhood cancer survivorship: Improving care and quality of life*. Washington, DC: The National Academies Press.
IOM. 2003c. *The future of the public health in the 21st century*. Washington, DC: The National Academies Press.
IOM. 2003d. *Large-scale biomedical science: Exploring strategies for future research*. Washington, DC: The National Academies Press.
IOM. 2006. *From cancer patient to cancer survivor: Lost in transition*. Washington, DC: The National Academies Press.
IOM. 2007. *Cancer biomarkers: The promises and challenges of improving detection and treatment a review of the Department of Defense program for breast cancer research*. Washington, DC: The National Academies Press.
IOM. 2008. *Cancer care for the whole patient: Meeting psychosocial health needs*. Washington, DC: The National Academies Press.
IOM. 2009. *Conflict of interest in medical research, education, and practice*. Washington, DC: The National Academies Press.
IOM. 2010a. *Evaluation of biomarkers and surrogate endpoints in chronic disease*. Washington, DC: The National Academies Press.
IOM. 2010b. *Hepatitis and liver cancer: A national strategy for prevention and control of hepatitis B and C*. Washington, DC: The National Academies Press.
IOM. 2010c. *A national cancer clinical trials system for the 21st century: Reinvigorating the NCI cooperative group program*. Washington, DC: The National Academies Press.
IOM. 2012. *Breast cancer and the environment: A life course approach*. Washington, DC: The National Academies Press.
IOM. 2013a. *Best care at lower cost: The path to continuously learning health care in America*. Washington, DC: The National Academies Press.
IOM. 2013b. *Delivering high-quality cancer care: Charting a new course for a system in crisis*. Washington, DC: The National Academies Press.
IOM. 2014. *Capturing social and behavioral domains and measures in electronic health records: Phase 2*. Washington, DC: The National Academies Press.
IOM. 2015. *Dying in America: Improving quality and honoring individual preferences near the end of life*. Washington, DC: The National Academies Press.
IQVIA. 2018. *Global oncology trends 2018*. Parsippany, NJ: IQVIA.
Isehunwa, O. O., E. L. Carlton, Y. Wang, Y. Jiang, S. Kedia, C. F. Chang, D. Fijabi, and S. S. Bhuyan. 2017. Access to employee wellness programs and use of preventive care services among US adults. *American Journal of Preventive Medicine* 53(6):854–865.
Juengst, E., M. L. McGowan, J. R. Fishman, and R. A. Settersten, Jr. 2016. From "personalized" to "precision" medicine: The ethical and social implications of rhetorical reform in genomic medicine. *Hastings Center Report* 46(5):21–33.
Kenya Ministry of Health. 2017. *National cancer control strategy 2017–2022*. Nairobi, Kenya: Ministry of Health, Kenya.
KFF and HRET (Kaiser Family Foundation and Health Research & Educational Trust). 2017. *Employer health benefits: 2017 summary of findings*. https://www.kff.org/report-section/ehbs-2017-summary-of-findings (accessed February 15, 2019).

Kopp, E., S. Lupkin, and E. Lucas. 2018. *Patient advocacy groups take in millions from drugmakers: Is there a payback?* https://khn.org/news/patient-advocacy-groups-take-in-millions-from-drugmakers-is-there-a-payback (accessed February 15, 2019).

Kutner, M., E. Greenburg, Y. Jin, and C. Paulsen. 2006. *The health literacy of America's adults: Results from the 2003 National Assessment of Adult Literacy.* NCES 2006-483. National Center for Education Statistics.

Kyzas, P. A., K. T. Loizou, and J. P. Ioannidis. 2005. Selective reporting biases in cancer prognostic factor studies. *Journal of the National Cancer Institute* 97(14):1043–1055.

Loeb, S. 2014. Guideline of guidelines: Prostate cancer screening. *BJU International* 114(3):323–325.

Love-Koh, J., A. Peel, J. C. Rejon-Parrilla, K. Ennis, R. Lovett, A. Manca, A. Chalkidou, H. Wood, and M. Taylor. 2018. The future of precision medicine: Potential impacts for health technology assessment. *Pharmacoeconomics* 36(12):1439–1451.

Major, A., and S. L. Stewart. 2009. Celebrating 10 years of the National Comprehensive Cancer Control Program, 1998 to 2008. *Preventing Chronic Disease* 6(4):A133.

Mango, V., Y. Bryce, E. A. Morris, E. Gianotti, and K. Pinker. 2018. Commentary ACOG practice bulletin July 2017: Breast cancer risk assessment and screening in average-risk women. *The British Journal of Radiology* 91(1090):20170907.

Mattke, S., H. Liu, J. Caloyeras, C. Y. Huang, K. R. Van Busum, D. Khodyakov, and V. Shier. 2013. Workplace wellness programs study: Final report. *RAND Health Quarterly* 3(2):7.

McCoy, M. S., M. Carniol, K. Chockley, J. W. Urwin, E. J. Emanuel, and H. Schmidt. 2017. Conflicts of interest for patient-advocacy organizations. *New England Journal of Medicine* 376(9):880–885.

McKeanna, M. A., E. Fabian, J. E. Hurley, B. T. McMahon, and S. L. West. 2007. Workplace discrimination and cancer. *Work* 29(4):313–322.

Merkel, P. A., M. Manion, R. Gopal-Srivastava, S. Groft, H. Jinnah, D. Robertson, and J. P. Krischer. 2016. The partnership of patient advocacy groups and clinical investigators in the rare diseases clinical research network. *Orphanet Journal of Rare Diseases* 11(1):66.

Microsoft News Center India. 2018. *Microsoft partners with SRL to expand AI network to detect cancer.* https://news.microsoft.com/en-in/microsoft-partners-with-srl-diagnostics-to-expand-ai-network-for-healthcare-to-pathology (accessed February 15, 2019).

Minari, J., K. B. Brothers, and M. Morrison. 2018. Tensions in ethics and policy created by national precision medicine programs. *Human Genomics* 12(1):22.

Moyer, V. A. 2012. Screening for prostate cancer: U.S. Preventive Services Task Force recommendation statement. *Annals of Internal Medicine* 157(2):120–134.

Murphy, D. G., T. Ahlering, W. J. Catalona, H. Crowe, J. Crowe, N. Clarke, M. Cooperberg, D. Gillatt, M. Gleave, S. Loeb, M. Roobol, O. Sartor, T. Pickles, A. Wootten, P. C. Walsh, and A. J. Costello. 2014. The Melbourne consensus statement on the early detection of prostate cancer. *BJU International* 113(2):186–188.

NASEM (National Academies of Sciences, Engineering, and Medicine). 2016a. *Ovarian cancers: Evolving paradigms in research and care.* Washington, DC: The National Academies Press.

NASEM. 2016b. *Biomarker tests for molecularly targeted therapies: Key to unlocking precision medicine.* Washington, DC: The National Academies Press.

NASEM. 2017. *Fostering integrity in research.* Washington, DC: The National Academies Press.

NASEM. 2018. *Making medicines affordable: A national imperative.* Washington, DC: The National Academies Press.

NASEM. 2019. *Reproducibility and replicability in science.* Washington, DC: The National Academies Press.

NCCN (National Comprehensive Cancer Network). 2018. *NCCN guidelines.* https://www.nccn.org/professionals/physician_gls/default.aspx (accessed February 15, 2019).

NCES (National Center for Education Statistics). 2018. *Elementary and secondary education.* https://nces.ed.gov/fastfacts/display.asp?id=372 (accessed February 15, 2019).
NCI (National Cancer Institute). 2018a. *National Cancer Act of 1937.* https://www.cancer.gov/about-nci/legislative/history/national-cancer-act-1937 (accessed February 15, 2019).
NCI. 2018b. *National Cancer Act of 1971.* https://www.cancer.gov/about-nci/legislative/history/national-cancer-act-1971 (accessed February 15, 2019).
NCI. 2019. *The Cancer Genome Atlas Program.* https://www.cancer.gov/about-nci/organization/ccg/research/structural-genomics/tcga (accessed February 15, 2019).
OMB (Office of Management and Budget). 2019. https://www.whitehouse.gov/omb (accessed February 15, 2019).
OPM (Office of Personnel Management). 2017. *Federal employees health benefits program flexibilities.* https://www.federalregister.gov/documents/2017/12/19/2017-27067/federal-employees-health-benefits-program-flexibilities (accessed February 15, 2019).
OPM. 2018a. *Policy: Work-life.* https://www.opm.gov/policy-data-oversight/worklife/health-wellness/#url=healthpromotion (accessed February 15, 2019).
OPM. 2018b. *Work-life: Health and wellness.* https://www.opm.gov/policy-data-oversight/worklife/health-wellness/#url=Tools-Resources (accessed February 15, 2019).
Ornstein, C., and K. Thomas. 2018. *What these medical journals don't reveal: Top doctors' ties to industry.* https://www.nytimes.com/2018/12/08/health/medical-journals-conflicts-of-interest.html (accessed February 15, 2019).
Prasad, V. 2016. Translation failure and medical reversal: Two sides to the same coin. *European Journal of Cancer* 52:197–200.
Qaseem, A., M. J. Barry, T. D. Denberg, D. K. Owens, and P. Shekelle. 2013. Screening for prostate cancer: A guidance statement from the clinical guidelines committee of the American college of physicians. *Annals of Internal Medicine* 158(10):761–769.
Rath, G. K., and A. K. Gandhi. 2014. National cancer control and registration program in India. *Indian Journal of Medical and Paediatric Oncology: Official Journal of Indian Society of Medical & Paediatric Oncology* 35(4):288.
Reuters. 2018. *Google, Tencent, Sequoia China join $15 million funding for pharma startup XtalPi.* https://www.reuters.com/article/us-google-tencent-ai/google-tencent-sequoia-china-join-15-million-funding-for-pharma-startup-xtalpi-idUSKBN1FD08W (accessed February 15, 2019).
Rochester, P. W., J. S. Townsend, L. Given, H. Krebill, S. Balderrama, and C. Vinson. 2010. Comprehensive cancer control: Progress and accomplishments. *Cancer Causes and Control* 21(12):1967–1977.
Rochester, P., D. S. Porterfield, L. C. Richardson, K. McAleer, E. Adams, and D. Holden. 2011. Piloting performance measurement for comprehensive cancer control programs. *Journal of Public Health Management and Practice* 17(3):275–282.
Romero, Y., D. Trapani, S. Johnson, Z. Tittenbrun, L. Given, K. Hohman, L. Stevens, J. S. Torode, M. Boniol, and A. M. Ilbawi. 2018. National cancer control plans: A global analysis. *The Lancet Oncology* 19(10):e546–e555.
Rose, S. L. 2013. Patient advocacy organizations: Institutional conflicts of interest, trust, and trustworthiness. *Journal of Law, Medicine & Ethics* 41(3):680–687.
Rose, S. L., J. Highland, M. T. Karafa, and S. Joffe. 2017. Patient advocacy organizations, industry funding, and conflicts of interest. *JAMA Internal Medicine* 177(3):344–350.
Rosso, R. J., and P. A. Davis. 2018. *Medicare and budget sequestration.* Washington, DC: Congressional Research Service.
Savoia, C., M. Volpe, G. Grassi, C. Borghi, E. Agabiti Rosei, and R. M. Touyz. 2017. Personalized medicine-a modern approach for the diagnosis and management of hypertension. *Clinical Science* 131(22):2671–2685.

Schoenfeld, J. D., and J. P. Ioannidis. 2012. Is everything we eat associated with cancer? A systematic cookbook review. *American Journal of Clinical Nutrition* 97(1):127–134.

Schwartz, L. M., and S. Woloshin. 2019. Medical marketing in the United States, 1997–2016. *JAMA* 321(1):80–96.

Schwartz, S. K. 2016. Silicon Valley's vision to transform healthcare. *Medical Economics* 93(1):40–43.

Siu, A. L. 2016. Screening for breast cancer: U.S. Preventive Services Task Force recommendation statement. *Annals of Internal Medicine* 164(4):279–296.

Smith, R. A., K. S. Andrews, D. Brooks, S. A. Fedewa, D. Manassaram-Baptiste, D. Saslow, O. W. Brawley, and R. C. Wender. 2018. Cancer screening in the United States, 2018: A review of current American Cancer Society guidelines and current issues in cancer screening. *CA: Cancer Journal for Clinicians* 68(4):297–316.

Snyderman, R. 2014. Personalized medicine 2014: Has healthcare been transformed? *Personalized Medicine* 11(4):365–368.

SSA (Social Security Administration). 2018. *Disability evaluation under social security* https://www.ssa.gov/disability/professionals/bluebook/13.00-NeoplasticDiseases-Malignant-Adult.htm (accessed February 15, 2019).

Statista. 2018a. *Alcohol tax revenue in the United States from 2000 to 2023* (in billion U.S. dollars).* https://www.statista.com/statistics/248952/revenues-from-alcohol-tax-and-forecast-in-the-us (accessed February 15, 2019).

Statista. 2018b. *Tobacco tax revenue and forecast in the United States from 2000 to 2023* (in billion U.S. dollars).* https://www.statista.com/statistics/248964/revenues-from-tobacco-tax-and-forecast-in-the-us (accessed February 15, 2019).

Stefan, D. C., A. M. Elzawawy, H. M. Khaled, F. Ntaganda, A. Asiimwe, B. W. Addai, S. Wiafe, and I. F. Adewole. 2013. Developing cancer control plans in Africa: Examples from five countries. *The Lancet Oncology* 14(4):e189–e195.

Stephens, S. 2018. *Employer-based clinics: A new practice setting*. https://www.healthecareers.com/article/healthcare-news/employer-based-clinics-a-new-practice-setting (accessed February 15, 2019).

Thomas, K. 2018. *Drug maker pays $360 million to settle investigation into charity kickbacks.* https://www.nytimes.com/2018/12/06/health/actelion-johnson-and-johnson-kickback-medicare.html (accessed February 15, 2019).

TINA (Truth in Advertising). 2018. *Cancer care: The deceptive marketing of hope*. https://www.truthinadvertising.org/cancer-care-the-deceptive-marketing-of-hope (accessed February 15, 2019).

Tomczak, K., P. Czerwinska, and M. Wiznerowicz. 2015. The Cancer Genome Atlas (TCGA): An immeasurable source of knowledge. *Contemporary Oncology* 19(1a):A68–A77.

Towers Watson. 2015. *High performing insights: Achieving high-performance employee plans with onsite health centers*. https://www.towerswatson.com/en-US/Insights/IC-Types/Survey-Research-Results/2015/06/achieving-high-performance-employee-plans-with-onsite-health-centers (accessed February 15, 2019).

Townsend, J. S., A. R. Moore, T. N. Mulder, and M. Boyd. 2015. What does a performance measurement system tell us about the national comprehensive cancer control program? *Journal of Public Health Management and Practice* 21(5):449–458.

UN (United Nations). 2017. *The sustainable development goals report 2017*. New York.

UNDP (United Nations Development Programme). 2013. *Addressing the social determinants of noncommunicable diseases*. New York: United Nations Development Programme.

USDA (Department of Agriculture). 2018a. *Agencies*. https://www.usda.gov/our-agency/agencies (accessed February 15, 2019).

USDA. 2018b. *Dietary guidelines*. https://www.cnpp.usda.gov/dietary-guidelines (accessed February 15, 2019).

USDA. 2018c. *National School Lunch. Program.* https://www.fns.usda.gov/nslp/national-school-lunch-program-nslp (accessed February 15, 2019).

USPSTF (U.S. Preventive Services Task Force). 2018. *Final recommendation statement: Prostate cancer: Screening.* https://www.uspreventiveservicestaskforce.org/Page/Document/RecommendationStatementFinal/prostate-cancer-screening1 (accessed June 20, 2019).

USPTO (Patent and Trademark Office). 2018. *Patents 4 Patients.* https://www.uspto.gov/patent/initiatives/patent-application-initiatives/patents-4-patients (accessed February 15, 2019).

Vater, L. B., J. M. Donohue, S. Y. Park, and Y. Schenker. 2016. Trends in cancer-center spending on advertising in the United States, 2005 to 2014. *JAMA Internal Medicine* 176(8):1214–1216.

Weinstein, J. N., E. A. Collisson, G. B. Mills, K. R. Shaw, B. A. Ozenberger, K. Ellrott, I. Shmulevich, C. Sander, and J. M. Stuart. 2013. The Cancer Genome Atlas pan-cancer analysis project. *Nature Genetics* 45(10):1113–1120.

WHO (World Health Organization). 2013. *Global action plan for the prevention and control of noncommunicable diseases 2013–2020.* Geneva, Switzerland: World Health Organization.

WHO. 2017. *Cancer prevention and control in the context of an integrated approach.* (WHA70.12).

World Bank. 2011. The growing danger of non-communicable diseases: Acting now to reverse course. Paper read at conference. Washington, DC: The World Bank Human Development Network.

Yang, W., J. H. Williams, P. F. Hogan, S. S. Bruinooge, G. I. Rodriguez, M. P. Kosty, D. F. Bajorin, A. Hanley, A. Muchow, and N. McMillan. 2014. Projected supply of and demand for oncologists and radiation oncologists through 2025: An aging, better-insured population will result in shortage. *Journal of Oncology Practice* 10(1):39–45.

Zullig, L. L., K. J. Sims, R. McNeil, C. D. Williams, G. L. Jackson, D. Provenzale, and M. J. Kelley. 2017. Cancer incidence among patients of the US Veterans Affairs health care system: 2010 update. *Military Medicine* 182(7):e1883–e1891.

3

Guiding the System of Cancer Control

When thinking about the cancer control system, it is helpful to consider it as being composed of multiple levels. At the societal level, there are multiple public- and private-sector agencies, institutions, organizations, and companies, which are all relatively independent agents, pursuing their missions and interests separately, sometimes in coordination or sometimes in conflict with one another. A second level includes social networks of individuals, families, and community groups, all again pursing their own aspirations and interests. At the biological level, cancer cells adapt to medical interventions with mutations that, in effect, help the cancer "learn" how to avoid or resist the intended consequences of the interventions. To the extent that there is any form of a "command level" in cancer control, it would consist of different administrative and political entities spread across society, making decisions about resource allocation and other policies. There is competition for resources not only within the cancer control system but also among entities in that system (e.g., cardiovascular or neurodegenerative diseases) and those outside it (e.g., environmental protection, space research, and naval resources).

This chapter introduces the concept of systems engineering, which is helpful in analyzing, developing, and making decisions concerning complex adaptive systems. In particular, the systems engineering approach requires and relies on the development of effective models of the system and its states. These models are then modified and improved under study to predict and respond to a system's likely behavior under various "futures." With that in mind, the chapter ultimately explores some essential ingredients for a planning and monitoring tool based on the principles of systems engineering that can be used to guide the cancer control system.

SYSTEMS ENGINEERING IN SOCIETY

The world today is full of complex systems: manufacturing systems, logistics systems, transportation systems, banking systems, and on and on. Most of them, like the cancer control system, developed over time with no overarching plan and no one entity in charge, so they tend to have many of the same challenges as the cancer control system, such as difficulty coordinating the different components, which are generally pursuing their own goals and interests. The discipline of systems engineering has evolved as a way of improving the performance of these and other large, complex systems.

Unlike most other engineering disciplines, which focus mainly on complicated systems that can be designed and understood by deconstructing them down into component parts and considering them independently, systems engineering is inherently holistic because the properties of the overall system depend on the interactions among the system's components, meaning that all those components must be considered at once. One of the primary tasks in systems engineering design and analysis, therefore, is understanding the component parts of a system and how they interact to produce the system's behavior. Such an analysis is generally the first step in working with a complex system, and it often involves creating a model-based simulation and testing it to see whether it accurately reproduces the system's behavior under different constraints and parameters. Once such a simulation has been constructed, it can be used to test how the system will respond to various stimuli and changes, which in turn makes it possible to learn how to guide—not "control"—the system to a certain degree.

A Case Scenario: The National Airspace System

As one example of systems engineering in action, consider the U.S. National Airspace System, a complex adaptive system that is part of the larger global transportation system. The system consists of the airspace over the United States and nearby bodies of water, the aircraft moving through that airspace, and all the facilities, technology, organizations, and people needed to make sure that these aircraft have safe journeys—airports, radar and other navigation equipment, weather detection and forecasting systems, air traffic controllers, communication equipment, landing systems, and so on (GAO, 2015) (see Figure 3-1).

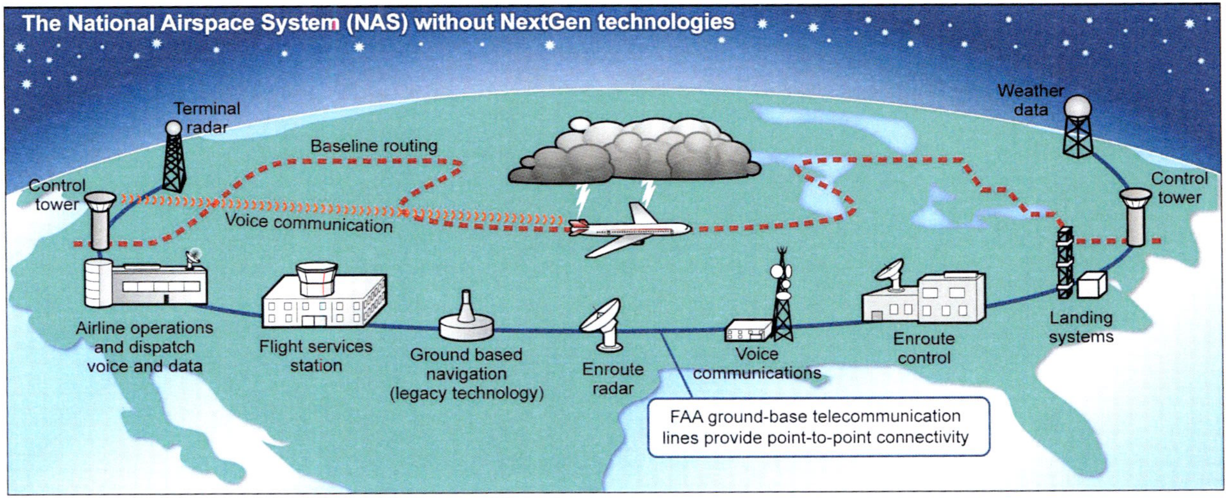

FIGURE 3-1 The National Airspace System, with and without NextGen technologies.
SOURCE: GAO-15-370.

continued

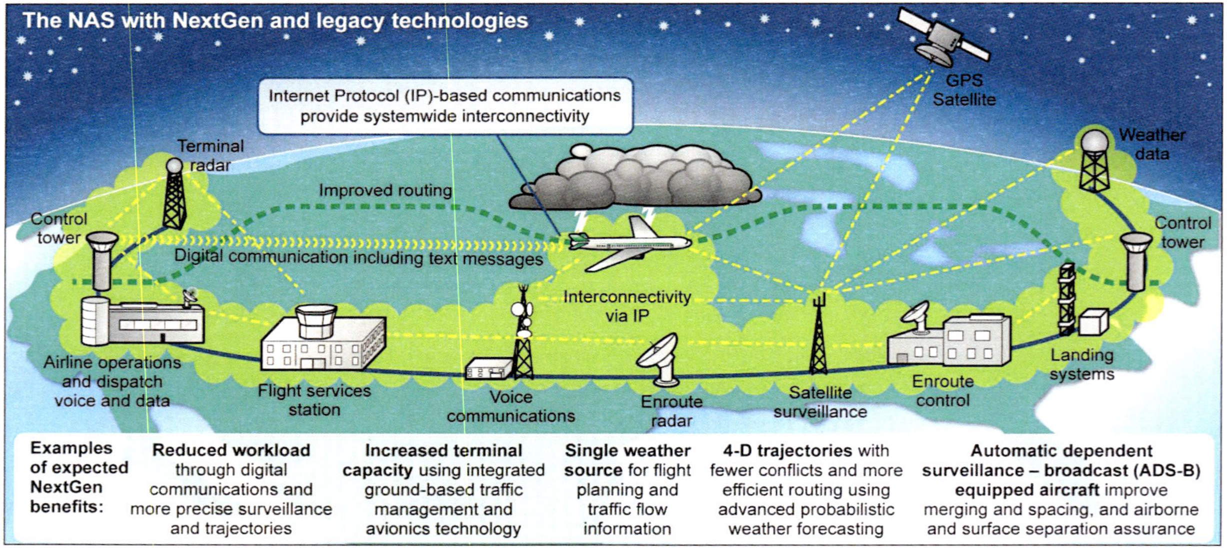

FIGURE 3-1 Continued

The National Airspace System is composed of many more different and smaller systems at work. Aircraft taking off from and landing at an airport with a control tower are the responsibility of a terminal radar approach control (TRACON). Once a plane climbs to about 18,000 feet, it is directed by one of 24 air route traffic control centers (ARTCCs), each responsible for a large section of the airspace over the United States (FAA, 2018). An aircraft is passed from one ARTCC to the next as it moves across the country until it approaches its destination and is handed off to the TRACON at that airport. Communication and coordination among the ARTCCs and TRACONs are crucial to monitoring all planes in U.S. airspace and to ensuring that they maintain safe distances from one another, horizontally and vertically.

The National Airspace System offers a clear example of the sort of communication and collaboration that must take place between the different components of a complex system if that system is to function effectively. In recent years, the National Airspace System has been modified with a set of so-called NextGen technologies (FAA, 2019a). A key improvement is the addition of satellite-based global positioning system (GPS) technologies that will be used to keep track of the planes (FAA, 2019b). Now, instead of relying on limited-range radar and handing off planes from one section to the next, the National Airspace System will be able to continuously monitor a plane's position across the entire country. With the GPS system, aircraft also receive precise information on the positions of other aircraft near them, improving safety. It is a good example of technological improvements being used to address some of the weaknesses in a system's operation—in this case, the limitations of using ground-based radar to keep track of thousands of planes as they fly across the country. It is worth noting that even with the installation of the NextGen technologies, the system remains complex. The improvements do not include any sort of hierarchical command system, which would be unworkable in a system this complex, but are simply making it possible for the different components of the system to all have access to more accurate information with which to make their decisions.

SYSTEMS APPROACHES IN CANCER CONTROL

The question that has prevailed in cancer control is how to achieve effectiveness and distributive equity while progressively diminishing the overall burden and costs. Thus, a promising path forward could be the adoption of a systems engineering approach—like that used with the National Airspace System—in which any sort of planning or development of strategies takes into account the entire system and its actions and interactions as a whole, instead of focusing on individual components.

This is not a novel conclusion, as many previous groups faced with similar problems—both in subsystems of cancer control and in other aspects of health and medicine—have concluded that systems analyses and approaches are the appropriate response (Hartwell et al., 2006; Huang et al., 2009; Leischow et al., 2008; Luke and Stamatakis, 2012).

A number of studies have applied—or attempted to apply—systems analysis and engineering to these individual subsystems. It is worth exploring this body of work, both because it offers lessons on how to apply systems thinking to the broad area of cancer control and also because any successful systems approach to cancer control will apply systems thinking not only to the entire system but also to its individual components considered as systems in their own right. It is also important to note that the systems engineering discussed in these various examples takes place at different levels, from the individual to the societal. Ultimately, any overarching approach to improving cancer control will have to act in a manner that is inclusive of all these different levels.

Clinical Care

Even relatively simple cancer cases can involve multiple components in the cancer care system: the patient, medical, surgical and radiation oncologists, pathologists, radiologists, hospitals, insurers, and so on. In the U.S. health care system, the involvement of so many different components may lead to less-than-effective care if coordination does not occur.

A recent case study illustrates this point (Trosman et al., 2016). The patient was a 32-year-old woman with breast cancer who was unemployed and enrolled in Medicaid. She was newly married and wanted to have children. The relevant parties were "the patient, the surgical office at a large hospital, the local oncology office, genetic counselors at the large hospital, an out-of-state genetic laboratory, a stand-alone fertility clinic, a local dental office, a local primary care provider, the psychosocial office at the large hospital, and the patient's Medicaid insurance" (p. 1102). The case study described four different situations in which the woman was failed by the health care system because of failure of the parties to work together effectively. For instance, although the woman wished to preserve her fertility, her treatment was begun without access to fertility preservation services. In addition, a failure to get the results of genetic testing before her surgery led the woman to undergo a different procedure than she would have if she had known the results ahead of time.

The case study concluded that the system of clinical cancer care needs to be modified to take into account the existence of "task interdependence"—that is, the ways in which the outcome of one task can be influenced by the outcome of another. Too often the different components of cancer care are treated as separate fragments with independent tasks, and improving cancer care depends on recognizing and allowing for the different ways that the components interact and, ultimately, finding ways to coordinate among those components.

Cancer Drug Delivery

Recent research in the realm of targeted drug delivery in cancer has also underscored the need for a systems approach. Drug targeting is best understood in the context of a system consisting of the tumor and the patient's surrounding tissues, the patient's body and health status overall, the drug or drugs being administered, the drug delivery system, and any other therapy modalities being used, such as radiation therapy (Dreher and Chilkoti, 2007). This integrated approach will be particularly important in the future because more treatments will depend on combinations of drugs in which the drug interactions are important and because emerging drug delivery technologies will make it possible to deliver drugs precisely to the tumor and avoid surrounding healthy tissue, but at the cost of having more complex delivery systems (Dreher and Chilkoti, 2007).

The development of the next generation of drug delivery systems will likely require effective interdisciplinary efforts of systems biologists, chemists, material scientists, bioengineers, pharmaceutical scientists, clinicians, and pharmacologists. The close collaboration required among these different participants will only be possible if the system is designed from the outset to recognize these interdependencies and collaboration patterns needed at different stages in the progression of delivery systems, from pre-clinical testing and clinical trials to post-approval observational studies used to generate "real-world evidence" of effectiveness. An analogy captures the point: "integration is key to getting all this to work on the therapeutic battlefield—integration of the warhead (drug) with the guidance system (targeting moiety) and with the rocket (the delivery vehicle)" (Dreher and Chilkoti, 2007). Therefore, a systems engineering approach is needed for the design of effective drug delivery systems.

Cancer Survivorship

Presently, there is substantial variation in the provision of cancer survivorship care services, and there is no standard way of evaluating that care. Because such an effort innately involves numerous participants, starting from the individual patient to insurance companies, coordinating resources and the necessary information most relevant to the patient is a perpetual challenge. A decade ago, survivorship care plans were proposed as a way to bring a basic degree of coordination (IOM, 2006), and have become an official recommendation by the Commission on Cancer and numerous other groups. A survivorship care plan typically contains important information about the cancer type, treatments received and their potential consequences, guidance for follow-up care, and supportive resources available for patients (IOM, 2006; McCabe et al., 2013). While survivorship care plans have primarily focused on informing patients of the effects of their treatments and improving communication between patients and clinicians, recent reports have also begun to consider their shortcomings, which include mixed effectiveness in improving health outcomes of survivors, and ways to improve survivorship care delivery (Jacobsen et al., 2018).

The Systems Engineering Initiative for Patient Safety (SEIPS) has sought to improve "health outcomes, quality of care delivery, transitions of care and coordination, usability, and implementation of health information technology, as well as managing a variety of health care activities, primary care workflows, and decision support" (Tevaarwerk et al., 2018, pp. 2–3). Applying the SEIPS method to cancer survivorship care would involve analyzing the various components of care for cancer survivors, their interactions, and the workflows in the system in order to identify where breakdowns and failures of communication occur and to develop methods to improve communication and coordination among those components. Using risk modeling for service applications, electronic health records, and the design and integration of different tasks performed by clinicians and the patients themselves, the recommendations that emerge from that method could enable improvements to the care process. While this is an example of the promise of systems engineering tools in survivorship care coordination, additional opportunities could be explored and tested to improve survivorship care delivery and improve the quality of life of survivors.

Patient Safety

The 2000 Institute of Medicine report *To Err Is Human* concluded that medical errors, which can result in patient harm or even death, are common in the health care system (IOM, 2000). Because cancer care is medically complex, it offers multiple points at which such errors can occur. A great deal of effort has been expended in exploring, classifying, and understanding the types and causes of these errors, with the goal of minimizing their occurrence. Once the various types of errors have been listed and explicated, the next step is to find ways to minimize the number and severity of the errors, and it is here that systems engineering can play a role in reducing the likelihood of miscommunication between two or more entities. Unfortunately, despite many calls for systems engineering partnership in the redesign of health and medical systems, there has been little movement in that direction, and medical errors remain a significant concern (Carayon and Wood, 2010).

Reducing Disparities

A conceptual systems model has been used to examine the factors contributing to health disparities across the cancer continuum. Three levels have been considered for those factors—distal, intermediate, and proximal (Paskett et al., 2016; Warnecke et al., 2008). The model suggests that the distal factors, which operate at the population level, are the fundamental causes of health disparities. This is because such factors influence individuals' health outcomes independently of the characteristics of individuals.

The distal influences include population-level social conditions, public policies, and institutional and other factors that stem from culture and social norms as well as socioeconomic status and the availability of health services. Intermediate influences include the immediate physical and social contexts as well as the social relationships in which the distal influences are experienced, such as the community or neighborhood. Proximal influences include individual genetic makeup; demographic factors such as age, health status, and race; and health behavior.

This model was applied in Delaware beginning in 2014 as part of an effort to reduce racial disparities in colorectal cancer (Grubbs et al., 2013). At the distal level of influence, the governor of Delaware legislated universal access to screening and treatment of colorectal cancer for all residents, with a statewide program that provided insurance coverage for these services for uninsured residents. At the intermediate level, the program relied extensively on nurses and care coordinators to engage and recruit underserved populations for screening as well as providing case management for patients with abnormal screening results. At the proximal level, the program collaborated with community organizations to reach African American communities and uninsured residents.

Data collected at the end of the program in 2009 indicated a reduction in colorectal cancer mortality and incidence rates among all residents of Delaware. Specifically, among African Americans, the incidence rate of colorectal cancer decreased from 66.9 per 100,000 to 44.3 per 100,000, and the mortality rate decreased from 31.2 per 100,000 to 18.0 per 100,000. Among whites, the incidence rate decreased from 58.2 per 100,000 to 43.2 per 100,000, and the mortality rate decreased from 19.5 per 100,000 to 16.9 per 100,000. In short, although the intervention lowered incidence and mortality rates among both African Americans and whites, the decreases were much greater for African Americans.

SYSTEMS ANALYSES AND SYSTEMATIC TRADE-OFFS

Making policies for complex adaptive systems is seldom straightforward. In the case of cancer control, for example, the simultaneous objectives would include maximizing survival rates, minimizing costs, maximizing quality-adjusted life years (QALYs), reducing side effects and errors, and addressing disparities and inequity. Different stakeholders have different objectives and value propositions. What payers value and prioritize may not be the same as the priorities for health care providers, commercial entities, or nonprofit organizations.

This section provides a case scenario of how a systems engineering approach can help inform policy analysis and decision making in a multilevel complex system. The goal of systems analysis is not to make the decision but to provide information about the trade-offs and help guide and achieve decision convergence on complex issues where the answers might change with time and context.

Multifactorial Analyses

Consider the case of vaccine development for cancer prevention and possibly therapy. In the past, pure health metrics (such as lives saved, infant mortality equivalents, and life years saved) or health economic measures such as cost-effectiveness (typically expressed in terms of dollars over QALYs or disability-adjusted life years [DALYs]) have been used to prioritize new vaccines for development. Cost–benefit analysis and its variant, cost-effectiveness analysis, have a rich history of guiding health policy decisions, but they also have widely recognized limits. For example, cost–benefit analysis typically poses complex ethical and political challenges by putting a specific monetary value on human life. Cost-effectiveness analysis, a close cousin of cost–benefit analysis, seeks to determine the incremental health benefits gained per incremental dollar invested. The resulting value, the incremental cost–effectiveness ratio, is compared against a cutoff value set by a decision maker (such as the £30,000-per-QALY figure used for evaluating medical interventions by the UK National Institute for Health and Care Excellence). The World Health Organization uses a cutoff of one to three times the per capita gross domestic product for cost-effectiveness calculated using DALYs (Marseille et al., 2014).

A major limitation of cost-effectiveness analyses is that a number of important considerations are left out of their calculation. These considerations include long-range issues, such as the spread of infection in a community over time; practical supply chain matters, such as a vaccine's temperature stability or how the vaccine fits within an immunization schedule; the herd immunity that can be achieved within a community if enough individuals are vaccinated; and higher level intergenerational issues, such as matters of equity (Phelps and Madhavan, 2017). Some recent efforts have attempted to "enhance" or "augment" cost-effectiveness analysis (Lakdawalla et al., 2018) by including such factors as scientific spillovers, the value of the hope that a disease might be cured, and gains in workforce productivity, but a major challenge remains: how to combine these various outcomes into a useful composite figure that takes into account both measurable and qualitative factors.

Those seeking to make policy decisions about cancer control face similar challenges. The traditional approach to valuing cancer control expenditures has been to use cost–benefit or cost-effectiveness analysis, but this leaves out many factors that are not easily quantified, such as the psychological stresses experienced by cancer survivors and their families or the societal costs of inequities in cancer incidence and treatment. Furthermore, different stakeholders will inevitably place different values on the various factors. Public health groups would likely place a higher value on different aspects of cancer control than cancer treatment clinics, both of which might differ from what a biopharmaceutical firm would most value. The National Institutes of Health, which is heavily focused on research, would place higher value on another set of activities, as would the Department of Agriculture or advocacy groups or a company like Google. Thus, ideally one would like to develop a systems analysis approach to evaluating cancer control activities that can weigh a variety of factors and can be personalized for different stakeholders.

A multi-attribute utility theory–based approach has been successfully prototyped in recent years for evaluating vaccine development. This approach to systems analysis makes it possible to include many different factors, each of which can have its own method of quantification. That quantification might be, for instance, a cost in dollars per QALY, a rating of public fear on a scale from 1 to 10, or even a yes/no value. Those values are all converted in such a way that their possible range is from 0 to 100, and in order to allow different vaccines to be compared, the same scales are used for all vaccines under consideration. Each vaccine is scored on each factor, that score is multiplied by a weighting value that reflects the importance of the factor, and the weighted scores are added up to get the vaccine's total score. That total reflects the value of the vaccine under a particular set of assumptions about how important each factor is; a different set of assumptions will lead to a different total score.

Performing a cost-effectiveness analysis of a vaccine—or a cancer treatment—requires, for example, assigning a value, or "utility," to various outcomes, such as being disease free and completely healthy or surviving the disease but with certain physical limitations. Such values can be estimated with data from population surveys or by expert panels, but they are far from objective. Additionally, some benefits of vaccines (or particular cancer control interventions) are next to impossible to assign value to. What is the value, for instance, of removing an individual's fear of contracting a disease or of decreasing the inequities in cancer rates and treatments?

One major benefit of multi-attribute systems analysis is that it allows policy makers and others to consider all these sorts of factors when considering which of various policies to choose. While traditional cost-effectiveness analyses have depended primarily on factors that can be easily quantified, multi-attribute systems analysis makes it possible to take into account the factors, such as issues of disparities, religious beliefs, or concerns pertaining to privacy and individual autonomy, that do influence policy making. The simple act of including such factors in a model can be enough to bring them to the attention of policy makers and enable those individuals to think about how to weigh these factors in their decisions.

A Case Illustration: Analysis of Alternatives for Cancer Vaccines

To illustrate how this systems analysis approach might be applied to an aspect of cancer control, an analysis was conducted on a completely hypothetical yet somewhat realistic scenario for prioritizing vaccines for human papillomavirus (HPV), a sexually acquired infection linked most commonly to cervical cancer (WHO, 2019). Trade-offs related to different HPV vaccines were calculated with SMART Vaccines, the Strategic Multi-Attribute Ranking Tool for Vaccines, a software system developed by the National Academies at the request of the Department of Health and Human Services (HHS) based on multi-criteria systems analysis—specifically, multi-attribute utility theory (Phelps et al., 2017).[1] SMART Vaccines was developed in response to the U.S. National Vaccine Plan issued by HHS as a dynamic, adaptive, priority-setting tool for use by a wide range of international stakeholders to systematically analyze (and compare) the options that are available and readily usable for vaccine-preventable illnesses.

The following case scenario was constructed, with the SMART Vaccines tool being used to consider three different kinds of hypothetical HPV vaccines for development or use in South Africa. More than 100 types of HPV exist, and at least 14 are known to cause cancer, particularly

[1] Detailed information concerning the technical details and use of the software and data sets can be found in (IOM, 2012, 2013; IOM and NAE, 2015). The software (v1.1) is downloadable from www.nap.edu/smartvaccines (accessed February 15, 2019).

cervical cancer, although some cancers of the vulva, vagina, penis, anus, head, and neck are also associated with HPV infection. In 2018, about 90 percent of new cervical cancer cases around the world—or 513,000 cases out of a total 570,000—were found in less developed countries (WHO, 2019). The prevalence of HPV in South Africa is known to be high. A recent survey of sexually active, HIV-negative women aged 16–22 years in two South African cities found that two-thirds of them were positive for HPV (Mbulawa et al., 2018). Vaccines against HPV 16 and HPV 18, the most prevalent cancer-causing types of HPV, have been developed, but they are not in widespread use in many countries around the world.

For the purposes of this hypothetical demonstration, the incidence of HPV in South Africa is estimated to be under 100 cases of HPV per 100,000, with a case fatality rate between 30 and 80 percent depending on the complications, which include cervical intraepithelial neoplasia and vulvar cancer. The complications differ in their severity and annual costs, which will be assumed to be between $300 and $5,500.

Now, consider a hypothetical government agency in South Africa involved in both research and product development (potentially through some private-sector partnership) trying to design a new vaccine or purchase a commercially available vaccine for HPV among three candidates, HPV-X, HPV-Y, and HPV-Z. All three candidates are intended for people over the age of 1 year and have an estimated effectiveness between 70 and 90 percent and coverage between 60 and 85 percent.

HPV-X is a single-dose vaccine offering a 25-year immunity and costing a hypothetical $13 per dose and $10 for administration per dose, and the vaccine development is expected to cost under $100 million. HPV-Y is a two-dose vaccine offering lifetime protection, costing $13 per dose, $12 for administrative expenses per dose, with development costs estimated between $100 million and $500 million. HPV-Z also confers lifetime immunity with a similar anticipated $100 million to $500 million development cost, and it costs $9 per dose and in administrative expenses, but it is a three-dose vaccine.

The user begins the analysis by selecting or defining the attributes of interest and then ranking them in order of importance. Of relevance to HPV priority setting are some factors selected from the collection of attributes in SMART Vaccines: cost-effectiveness (cost per QALYs); demonstration of new production platforms (this includes scientific spillovers or use of existing manufacturing approaches to produce new vaccines); potential litigation barriers beyond usual (an issue that comes to fore with HPV vaccines); fitting into the existing immunization schedule (given the comparison involving multi-dose vaccines); and raising public health awareness of HPV-related cancers (a potential collateral benefit associated with promoting safe sex practices). Next, the user determines the weights to assign to the different attributes. The process is assisted by SMART Vaccines, which offers a suggested weighting that is based on the average of all the different possible sets of weights that are consistent with the user's ranking of the attributes. These initial weights can be adjusted by the user with slider bars provided by SMART Vaccines. In this HPV scenario, the initial suggested weights are used. Among the attributes in this example, cost-effectiveness is the highest ranked (with a 46 percent weight), and the attribute of the vaccine raising public health awareness is lowest ranked (with a 4 percent weight) (see Figure 3-2).

If one were to conduct a pure cost-effectiveness analysis—setting additional attributes selected for demonstration at 0—of these three HPV vaccine candidates, they are comparably cost-effective, with each achieving the high score of 100 through its cost savings or health benefits. HPV-X produces $101 per QALY, and HPV-Y and HPV-Z produce a net savings (indicated by negative) of $493 per QALY, each essentially tied at a SMART Score of 100. (The range of scores is typically 0 to 100, with 0 representing a vaccine that has no effect and 100 corresponding to a vaccine that is highly successful on all the attributes under consideration. The scores may go beyond 100 [better than the envisioned best-case scenario] or below zero [worse than the envisioned worst-case scenario] depending on their superiority or inferiority of their performance.) These numbers can easily be altered, with transparency, by changing the disease burden and vaccine profile according to the simulated or real circumstances. These changes can be made in a manner that makes it clear to the user why certain changes have occurred—a feature that is otherwise not so easily available in standard cost-effectiveness analyses, which do not capture the broader complexity of cancers and their impact on specific programs or larger aspects of social policy.

Next, the other attributes in SMART Vaccines are brought into the analysis; these include domains across health, programmatic, public concerns, and scientific and business considerations as well as intangible values. According to this hypothetical scenario, the single-dose HPV-X readily fits into the immunization schedule, does not contain potential litigation barriers beyond usual, and raises public health awareness but does not beneficially demonstrate new production platforms. HPV-Y is largely similar to HPV-X except that it requires two doses and, because of this additional dose, may pose additional litigation issues, something that also is the case with HPV-Z, the three-dose vaccine. HPV-Z offers novelty or efficiency in production methods and, because of multiple doses, does not readily fit into any existing immunization schedules, thus simultaneously presenting scientific advantages but logistical challenges. The resulting SMART Scores based on these entries are shown in Figure 3-3. Despite multiple doses and potential litigation barriers, the HPV-Z

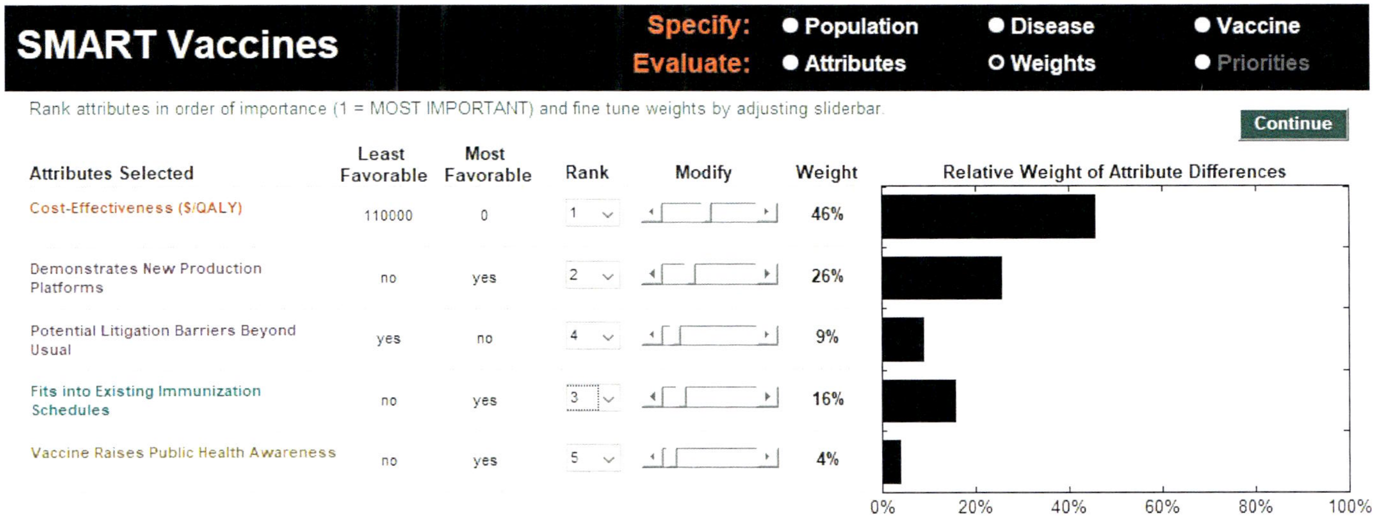

FIGURE 3-2 Multi-attribute selection for systems analysis using SMART Vaccines. Attributes are selected and ranked with an initial suggestion of weights provided by the software consistent with the user's rank ordering alterable using slider bars. Five attributes of relevance are shown here for a demonstration using three hypothetical HPV vaccines for use in South Africa.

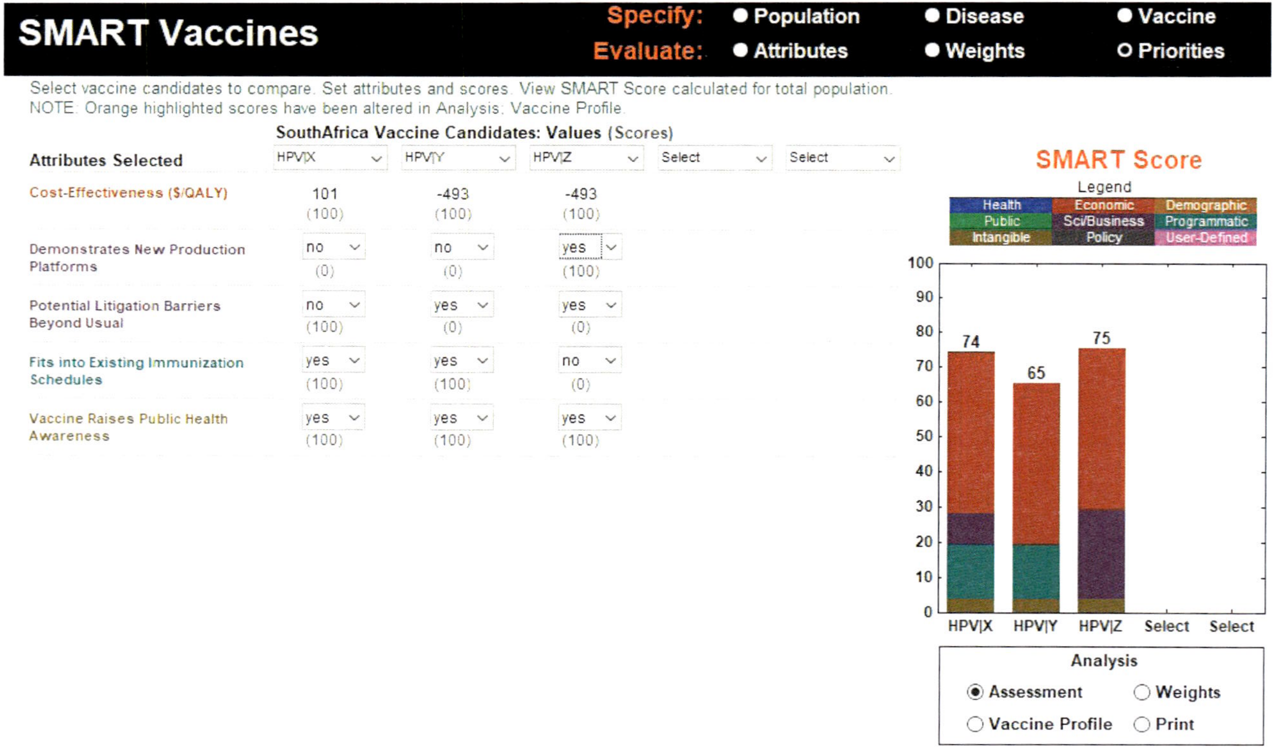

FIGURE 3-3 Systems analyses of product features and trade-offs using five attributes comparing three hypothetical human papillomavirus vaccines (HPV-X, HPV-Y, HPV-Z) for use in South Africa. Color coding denotes the contribution of individual attribute segment (health, programmatic, scientific and business, public concerns, and intangible values) to the final SMART Scores.

vaccine scores higher than HPV-X (at 74) and HPV-Y (at 65). With changes in weights, the results will naturally change, and sensitivity analysis can be conducted (using the "vaccine profile" button in SMART Vaccines) to reverse engineer a product profile to improve the performance of a candidate either, for example, through boosting coverage (a programmatic matter) or effectiveness (a scientific matter) or through cost reduction (an administrative and industrial manufacturing matter) or, ultimately, dosage alteration. One could conceivably work toward developing desirable hybrid attributes (for example, imagining a two-dose HPV-Z) or using a two-dose HPV-Y and supplementing it with additional social, scientific, or policy tools to increase its performance.

The results create an important discussion opportunity among participants on why a particular vaccine candidate may be scientifically better, economically preferred, or more politically feasible over another. These kinds of discussions might be particularly valuable in an interagency setting or a national or international advisory group with individuals and institutions bringing varying perspectives on issues of common interests. It is possible to envision and apply multi-criteria decision support to many aspects of population health and medicine, especially cancer control. The next section explores that prospect.

BUILDING A MULTI-LEVEL MODEL

The preceding multi-criteria systems analysis shows that it is possible to construct a decision-support model that captures an important aspect of cancer control—deciding on a vaccine strategy—and allows policy makers to consider a variety of criteria in choosing which direction to go. A key aspect of multi-criteria approaches is that it makes it possible to weigh different strategies by comparing the outcomes of those strategies on a number of different measures chosen by the user. Importantly, multi-criteria approaches could also enable an expanded analysis of types of outcomes—economic, clinical, scientific, and otherwise—through different measures. Five such factors are illustrated in Figure 3-4: the strength of the evidence, the magnitude of the problem, the actions taken, barriers and facilitators, and the strategies across participant groups to determine which activities need to be improved, revamped, or terminated (Norton et al., 2018).

One could envision a similar—albeit much more complicated—"model of models" that captured the entire cancer control system and similarly made it possible to compare the outcomes of different sets of strategies as evaluated by various measures. How would one go about creating such a model? The following is one possible approach.

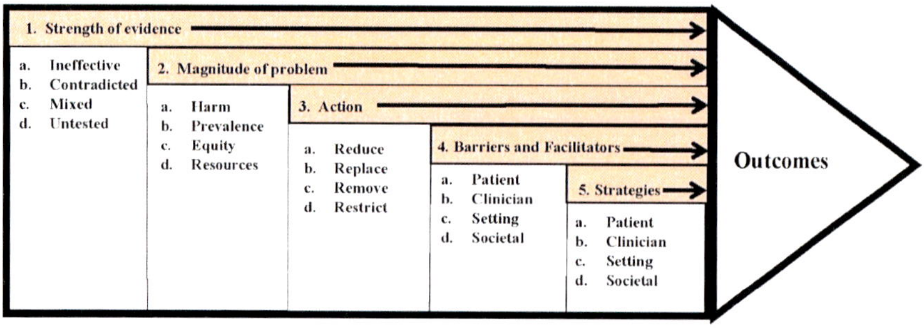

FIGURE 3-4 A multi-criteria outcomes framework.
SOURCE: Adapted from Norton et al., 2018.

The Levels of Cancer Control

As discussed earlier, the cancer control system spans a number of levels, and thus any model of the cancer control system will inevitably be a multi-level model with a combination of individual models that capture various aspects of the overall system. In recent years, a number of frameworks for modeling complex social systems, such as higher education, medical services, and population health, have been proposed (Rouse et al., 2019). One conceptual description centers on integrating several models that had been suggested for understanding the roles of various factors—social, psychological, political, economic, and biological—in determining health and health disparities (Kaplan, 2004). This concept follows that general pattern by describing a multi-level model of cancer control. In particular, the general model proposed here has four levels, each of which can be modeled separately and then linked with the others to produce a full model (Madhavan et al., 2018) (see Figure 3-5).

The levels of the model are population ecosystem, or society; system structure, or organization; delivery operations, or processes; and service interactions, or people. Modeling each of these levels is a separate challenge. The organizational level, for example, is described by the microeconomics of resource allocation, with decision theory and behavioral economics used to model the behavior of individuals involved in the organizations. The society level is described mainly by macroeconomics. In use, the model would be set up to be interactive so that a user could change the values of various parameters and observe the results; those results would typically be shown through some sort of visualization that would allow the user to make sense of the complex behavior of the system.

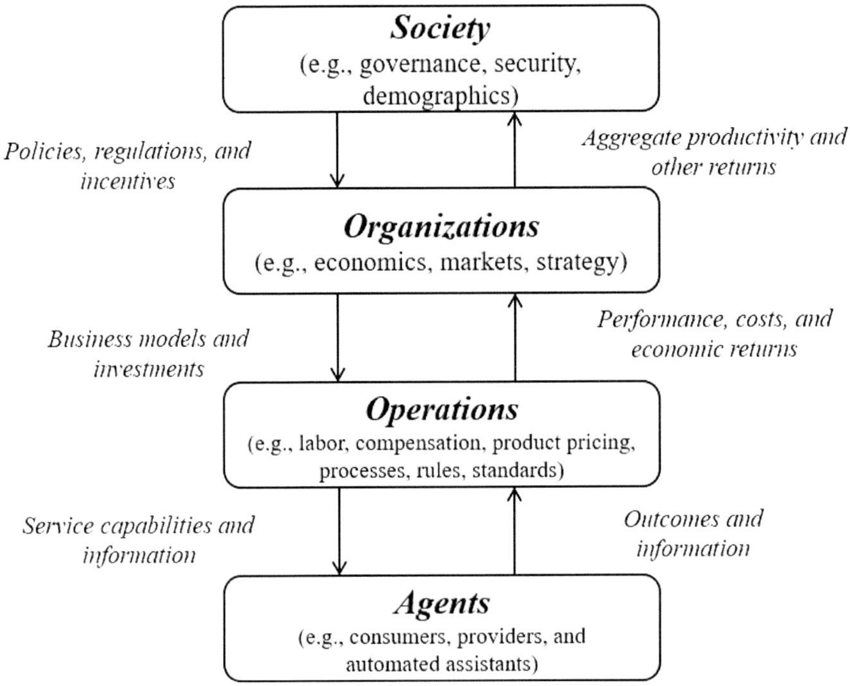

FIGURE 3-5 A multi-level abstraction of a population health system architecture relating to the flow and compatibility of information from society to individual agents, and vice versa. Additional arrows showing flows of influences across layers have been omitted for visual clarity.
SOURCE: Madhavan et al., 2018.

A Family of Models

A model of the U.S. cancer control system would serve the same sort of purpose as a multi-criteria, multi-level model, just on a much larger scale. That is, it would allow stakeholders to see the likely outcome of various competing options, and, in so doing, it would help stakeholders clarify their values and priorities.

In building such a model, it will be possible—and desirable—to draw on the large number of existing models of various aspects of the cancer control system. For example, the researchers who are part of the Cancer Intervention and Surveillance Modeling Network (CISNET) have built a number of models predicting the outcomes of specific types of cancer depending on various factors, such as screening rates or the development of new treatments. One group of CISNET researchers, for example, created a model that projected the rates of smoking over the next 50 years and used that to predict what the annual incidence rates and death rates from lung cancer will be up through 2065 (Jeon et al., 2018). There are CISNET models for certain types of cancer. They can be used to predict incidence rates and deaths (among other factors), given the appropriate inputs, such as individual behaviors (smoking, vaccination), technological factors (the development of new treatments or drugs), and economic factors (the cost of treatment, for example).

There are many other types of existing models that could also be used in building a model of the U.S. cancer control system. Various population-level models can be used to project different aspects of the population in coming years, such as the numbers of people and their ages living in rural, suburban, and urban areas in 2040 or the rates of obesity by age and sex in 2025. There are also models that can forecast rates of various types of relevant behavior, such as the vaccination rates for different groups of people or the rates of compliance with recommended treatment follow-up. While it is not likely that every important aspect of the cancer control system has been modeled or has a model that can be applied to it, that is true for most of them.

Technical challenges will certainly arise when one starts to combine these models to create, say, one model or a suite of linked core models of the entire cancer control system. To begin with, there is wide variation in how detailed the models are and how well they work. Some are very basic models designed to capture large-scale trends, while others have much more detailed projections. Some are well validated in a variety of settings, while others have not been tested nearly so thoroughly. A key challenge will come from the variations in how the different models define the variables they use and the data they rely on. If the different models are to fit together to form a single model of the cancer control system, they will all need to use the same variables and rely on the same data, which means that it will be necessary to first settle on the data standards that will be used for the model and then modify the individual models to use those standards. Once that is done, the individual models will need to be verified and validated with the new standards and data formats. The resulting family of models will provide the "raw materials" that will be assembled to create the overarching model of the cancer control system.

As the models are combined, new capabilities will appear. For example, a behavioral model that predicts the effectiveness of antismoking campaigns in getting people to stop smoking could be combined with an epidemiological model of lung cancer as a function of smoking rates to make it possible to see what effects an increase in funding for antismoking campaigns would have on lung cancer rates over the next several decades. Or projections of immigration from countries where the smoking rate is higher could be used to sharpen the forecasts of how many people living in the United States are likely to smoke in 2030 or 2040.

The perceptive reader will have noticed a disconnect between this description of a family of models used to capture the cancer control system and the concept of cancer control being a complex adaptive system, which by its very nature cannot be decomposed into component parts that can be analyzed individually. How then could such a family of models accurately capture the behavior of the cancer control system?

The answer has several parts. First, the fact that cancer control is a complex adaptive system does not imply that none of its component parts can be modeled individually. They can—as long as it is known what the inputs from the rest of the system are. The complexity arises because of the feedback loops among the components: component A affects component B affects component C, which in turn affects component M, which links back to component A. So whatever model one designs will have to accurately reflect how the different components interact with and affect one another, but that is a separate issue from whether the individual components can be effectively modeled. In addition, there are likely to be cases where the interactions between components, while present, are insignificant enough that they can be ignored by the model or added in as a correction factor toward the end of a simulation run. And in cases where the interaction between components is particularly strong, it would likely make sense to model them together instead of modeling them separately and later adding the interactions.

In short, while the interactions between components will certainly need to be captured in the overall model, a family of models that capture individual elements of the cancer control system will form the foundation of the overall model.

GUIDANCE SYSTEMS FOR CANCER CONTROL

The ultimate goal of assembling such a family of models will be to create a system that can be used not just to make predictions about the performance of the cancer control system under various scenarios but ultimately to guide the cancer control system. As noted earlier, the choice of the verb "guide" instead of a word like "control" or "direct" is deliberate. As a complex adaptive system, cancer control cannot be directed. It can, however, be "influenced" or "guided" in such a way that it moves in a desired direction—becoming more efficient, for example, or more equitable. Developing such a guidance system will be a major undertaking (and is far beyond the scope of this report to provide a construction blueprint). However, it is possible to discuss what some of the system's characteristics and features might be.

A Systems Architecture for Cancer Control

The first step must be to understand the present system, its principal components, and their interactions. These components will include various governmental bodies and agencies that set cancer-related policy, research and funding organizations, clinical research entities at hospitals and universities, the biopharmaceutical and device industry, the health insurance industry, professional organizations, individual patients and their families, and advocacy groups, among others. Any model that captures this system will be exceedingly complicated and will not decompose into separate pieces that can be understood in isolation. It will include multiple subsystems—hospitals and clinicians, researchers, the insurance industry, government regulators, patient advocacy and support groups, and biopharmaceutical companies—and it will include multiple levels, from the biological to the societal.

Some of the concepts for such a multi-level modeling effort already exist. A 2012 article, for example, identified seven levels at which cancer care could be influenced: the individual patients, family and social supports, the clinical team, the clinical practice setting, the local community, the state health policy environment, and the national health policy environment (Taplin et al., 2012). These are different from, but closely related to, the four levels described earlier that are envisioned for use in analyzing and advancing the cancer control system.

Planning and Policy Setting

With the model established, the next step will be to create a simulation that can mimic the behavior of the system and then test that simulation for accuracy. One way to do that is to look to the recent past and see whether the system can "predict" what happened or "forecast" possible futures. Can it, for instance, accurately predict the response of the entire system to the introduction of a new technology, such as an effective drug? Can it accurately model the behavior of hospitals and clinics when a major change in insurance policies occurs?

A main purpose of the simulation is to show how the performance of the system changes as a result of specific modifications. The simulation requires continual updates with the most recent data so that it reflects current information. This monitoring will make it possible to detect trends and to test the accuracy of forecasts. If the simulation is to be useful in predicting how various changes will affect the system's performance, it should certainly be able to predict outcomes in the near term without any major changes in the system. In addition, the system should be able to learn by comparing its forecasts with what actually happens. Figure 3-6

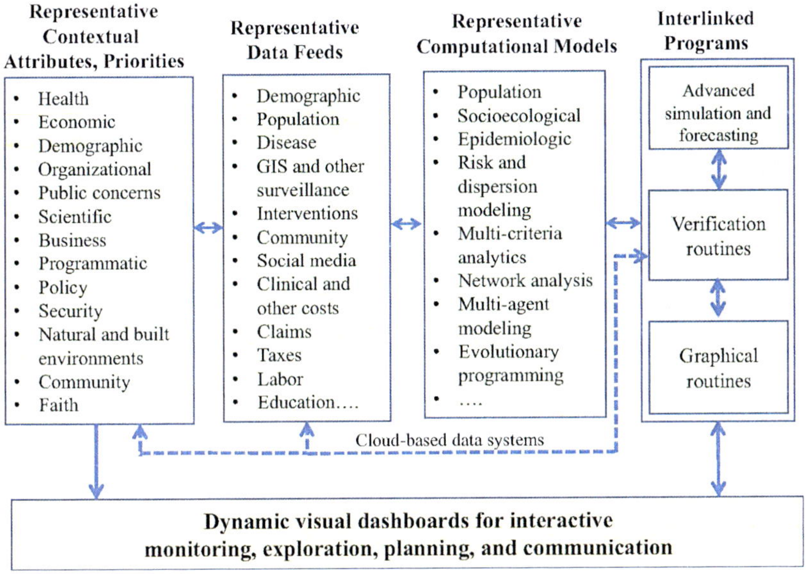

FIGURE 3-6 A generic population health systems architecture for visual monitoring, exploration, planning, and communication strategies with potential use for cancer control analyses.
SOURCE: Madhavan et al., 2018.

shows a generic population health systems architecture, customizable for cancer control efforts, that blends contextual attributes and priorities with necessary data feeds from different channels operated on by different computational models that ultimately produce a dynamic visual dashboard to track, plan for, and initiate joint action among multiple constituents.

Construction of such a population health systems architecture will make it possible to run, evaluate, and compare different scenarios and outcomes to aid in policy making. For example, what will happen to cancer rates over the next two decades under different funding allocations between prevention efforts and complex treatment regimens with or without constraints on the use and cost of treatment for different tumor classes and subtypes?

One of the most useful aspects of such a system architecture would be the ability to see what the collective demands are at any particular point and what happens when coordinated changes are made to various components of the cancer control system in response to those demands or in advance of any potential changes in health. There is a growing agreement across various stakeholders that, to be effective, changes made to a system such as cancer control will need to be made at multiple levels simultaneously (Taplin et al., 2012), but there currently is no capability of determining what effects a set of changes carried out at multiple levels is likely to have.

Finally, once such a comprehensive model of models has been developed, policy makers could use it to zero in on a set of changes necessary to guide the cancer control system in a desired direction. These could be changes in the allocation of funding among research, public health initiatives, training of medical personnel, and so on; they could be new regulations covering hospitals and medical practices or insurance coverage; they could be modifications to pharmaceutical patent policies; or they could be any other changes the government could initiate that would affect the cancer control system. Once the changes and the related assumptions had been put in place, the system would monitor the effects of those changes and use that feedback to sharpen future simulations and develop a learning process.

FINDINGS

Finding 3-1: *Looking ahead, complex systems analytics made possible by the convergence of modern computational technologies—including biotechnologies, nanotechnologies, communication, social media, cognitive, sensor technologies, and other systems engineering tools—could materially amplify new insights, capabilities, and competencies necessary for advancing cancer control and potentially reducing costs for the United States.*

Finding 3-2: *Systems engineering tools have been effectively applied to design, guide, influence, and improve complex adaptive systems in multiple industrial and other settings across society. Some previous analyses involving clinical care and survivorship services have recognized the role of systems engineering approaches to offer both operational insights and prospects for effective cancer control.*

Finding 3-3: *Multi-criteria systems analyses offer promise to transcend the narrow analytical tools used across different aspects of health and medical policies and could support individual and group decision making at multiple levels, including critically reviewing which activities need to be initiated, improved, scaled, or discontinued as cancer control efforts evolve.*

Finding 3-4: *Developing a guidance system to fully understand the influences and impacts on a national cancer control plan requires a comprehensive planning and monitoring tool or a set of linked tools able to integrate different data and* *perspectives, blend modeling and simulation capabilities, and produce dynamic visuals for interactive monitoring, exploration, planning, and communication.*

REFERENCES

Carayon, P., and K. E. Wood. 2010. Patient safety—the role of human factors and systems engineering. *Studies in Health Technology and Informatics* 153:23–46.

Dreher, M. R., and A. Chilkoti. 2007. Toward a systems engineering approach to cancer drug delivery. *Journal of the National Cancer Institute* 99(13):983–985.

FAA (Federal Aviation Administration). 2018. *Administrator's fact book: December 2018.* https://www.faa.gov/news/media/2018_Administrators_Fact_Book.pdf (accessed February 15, 2019).

FAA. 2019a. *Modernization of U.S. Airspace.* https://www.faa.gov/nextgen (accessed February 15, 2019).

FAA. 2019b. *Performance based navigation in the operation.* https://www.faa.gov/nextgen/how_nextgen_works/new_technology/pbn/in_depth (accessed February 15, 2019).

GAO (Government Acountability Office). 2015. *Air traffic control: FAA needs a more comprehensive approach to address cybersecurity as agency transitions to NextGen.* GAO-15-370. April. Washington, DC: U.S. Government Accountability Office.

Grubbs, S. S., B. N. Polite, J. Carney Jr, W. Bowser, J. Rogers, N. Katurakes, P. Hess, and E. D. Paskett. 2013. Eliminating racial disparities in colorectal cancer in the real world: It took a village. *Journal of Clinical Oncology* 31(16):1928.

Hartwell, L., D. Mankoff, A. Paulovich, S. Ramsey, and E. Swisher. 2006. Cancer biomarkers: A systems approach. *Nature Biotechnology* 24(8):905.

Huang, T. T., A. Drewnowski, S. K. Kumanyika, and T. A. Glass. 2009. A systems-oriented multilevel framework for addressing obesity in the 21st century. *Preventing Chronic Disease* 6(3).

IOM (Institute of Medicine). 2000. *To err is human: Building a safer health system.* Washington, DC: National Academy Press.

IOM. 2006. *From cancer patient to cancer survivor: Lost in transition.* Washington, DC: The National Academies Press.

IOM. 2012. *Ranking vaccines: A prioritization framework: Phase I: Demonstration of concept and a software blueprint.* Washington, DC: The National Academies Press.

IOM. 2013. *Ranking vaccines: A prioritization software tool: Phase II: Prototype of a decision-support system.* Washington, DC: The National Academies Press.

IOM and NAE (Institute of Medicine and National Academy of Engineering). 2015. *Ranking vaccines: Applications of a prioritization software tool: Phase III: Use case studies and data framework.* Washington, DC: The National Academies Press.

Jacobsen, P. B., A. P. DeRosa, T. O. Henderson, D. K. Mayer, C. S. Moskowitz, E. D. Paskett, and J. H. Rowland. 2018. Systematic review of the impact of cancer survivorship care plans on health outcomes and health care delivery. *Journal of Clinical Oncology* 36(20):2088–2100.

Jeon, J., T. R. Holford, D. T. Levy, E. J. Feuer, P. Cao, J. Tam, L. Clarke, J. Clarke, C. Y. Kong, and R. Meza. 2018. Smoking and lung cancer mortality in the united states from 2015 to 2065: A comparative modeling approach. *Annals of Internal Medicine* 169(10):684–693.

Kaplan, G. A. 2004. What's wrong with social epidemiology, and how can we make it better? *Epidemiologic Reviews* 26(1):124–135.

Lakdawalla, D. N., J. A. Doshi, L. P. Garrison, C. E. Phelps, A. Basu, and P. M. Danzon. 2018. Defining elements of value in health care—a health economics approach: An ISPOR special task force report [3]. *Value in Health* 21(2):131–139.

Leischow, S. J., A. Best, W. M. Trochim, P. I. Clark, R. S. Gallagher, S. E. Marcus, and E. Matthews. 2008. Systems thinking to improve the public's health. *American Journal of Preventive Medicine* 35(2):S196–S203.

Luke, D. A., and K. A. Stamatakis. 2012. Systems science methods in public health: Dynamics, networks, and agents. *Annual Review of Public Health* 33:357–376.

Madhavan, G., C. E. Phelps, W. B. Rouse, and R. Rappuoli. 2018. Vision for a systems architecture to integrate and transform population health. *Proceedings of the National Academy of Sciences* 115(50):12595–12602.

Marseille, E., B. Larson, D. S. Kazi, J. G. Kahn, and S. Rosen. 2014. Thresholds for the cost-effectiveness of interventions: Alternative approaches. *Bulletin of the World Health Organization* 93:118–124.

Mbulawa, Z. Z., C. van Schalkwyk, N.-C. Hu, T. L. Meiring, S. Barnabas, S. Dabee, H. Jaspan, J.-M. Kriek, S. Z. Jaumdally, and E. Muller. 2018. High human papillomavirus (HPV) prevalence in South African adolescents and young women encourages expanded HPV vaccination campaigns. *PLoS ONE* 13(1):e0190166.

McCabe, M. S., S. Bhatia, K. C. Oeffinger, G. H. Reaman, C. Tyne, D. S. Wollins, and M. M. Hudson. 2013. American Society of Clinical Oncology statement: Achieving high-quality cancer survivorship care. *Journal of Clinical Oncology* 31(5):631.

Norton, W. E., D. A. Chambers, and B. S. Kramer. 2018. Conceptualizing de-implementation in cancer care delivery. *Journal of Clinical Oncology* 37(2):93–96.

Paskett, E., B. Thompson, A. S. Ammerman, A. N. Ortega, J. Marsteller, and D. Richardson. 2016. Multilevel interventions to address health disparities show promise in improving population health. *Health Affairs* 35(8):1429–1434.

Phelps, C. E., and G. Madhavan. 2017. Using multicriteria approaches to assess the value of health care. *Value in Health* 20(2):251–255.

Phelps, C. E., G. Madhavan, and B. Gellin. 2017. Planning and priority setting for vaccine development and immunization. *Vaccine* 35:A50–A56.

Rouse, W. B., K. M. Pepe, and M. M. Johns. 2019. Population health as a network of services: Integration of health, education, and social services. *Handbook of Service Science* 2:589–618.

Taplin, S. H., R. Anhang Price, H. M. Edwards, M. K. Foster, E. S. Breslau, V. Chollette, I. Prabhu Das, S. B. Clauser, M. L. Fennell, and J. Zapka. 2012. Introduction: Understanding and influencing multilevel factors across the cancer care continuum. *Journal of the National Cancer Institute. Monographs* 2012(44):2–10.

Tevaarwerk, A. J., J. R. Klemp, G. J. van Londen, B. W. Hesse, and M. E. Sesto. 2018. Moving beyond static survivorship care plans: A systems engineering approach to population health management for cancer survivors. *Cancer* 124(22):4292–4300.

Trosman, J. R., R. C. Carlos, M. A. Simon, D. L. Madden, W. J. Gradishar, A. B. Benson III, B. D. Rapkin, E. S. Weiss, I. F. Gareen, and L. I. Wagner. 2016. Care for a patient with cancer as a project: Management of complex task interdependence in cancer care delivery. *Journal of Oncology Practice* 12(11):1101–1113.

Warnecke, R. B., A. Oh, N. Breen, S. Gehlert, E. Paskett, K. L. Tucker, N. Lurie, T. Rebbeck, J. Goodwin, and J. Flack. 2008. Approaching health disparities from a population perspective: The National Institutes of Health Centers for Population Health and Health Disparities. *American Journal of Public Health* 98(9):1608–1615.

WHO (World Health Organization). 2019. *Human papillomavirus (HPV) and cervical cancer.* https://www.who.int/news-room/fact-sheets/detail/human-papillomavirus-(hpv)-and-cervical-cancer (accessed February 15, 2019).

4

A Path to Transformation

When one examines the approaches in cancer control to this point in time, the most obvious characteristic—besides the size and scale—is the complexity. The system of cancer control in the United States—and to some extent worldwide—has developed unevenly over time, with contributions from different people and groups focusing on various aspects of cancer. Clinical and biomedical researchers experimented with different approaches to preventing, detecting, and treating the disease, gradually settling on current practices. Biomedical scientists and engineers set out to understand the biological underpinnings of cancer in hopes of finding insights into its prevention and treatment. Biopharmaceutical companies searched for and developed drugs that would be effective against cancer while confronting the market realities of high risks and failures. Population health specialists sought to identify and modify environmental and behavioral risks that were contributing to cancer. Federal agencies, state legislatures, and local governments provided plans and regulations intended to direct cancer control efforts. Advocacy groups and professional associations added their voices, driving certain policies and approaches to help individuals with cancer or at risk of cancer.

The result has been a sprawling, mostly uncoordinated system that falls far short of the ideal in a variety of ways. There is, for example, no uniform way to examine the expenditures or to assess the various research outputs to determine reliable evidence for cancer control, decide on priorities, and then move forward in concert with those priorities. Ideally, for instance, one would want research funders and policy makers to have a way to determine the best allocation of resources among the various prevention, treatment, or other efforts and to push the system toward that allocation; there is no way to do that today. Even if it was known how to do this precisely and judiciously, the fragmentation of the current system and its constituent processes and interests do not permit the kind of resource analyses and allocation needed to maximally benefit patients and society at large. More generally, it would be desirable to have an established method for studying the various trade-offs that exist in cancer control, to help decide which trade-offs are in the best interests of population health.

Another major shortcoming of the current cancer control efforts is the presence and possible perpetuation of wide disparities across populations. Not only do certain cancers affect some populations at greater rates than others, but the care provided for certain populations is often less timely and less effective. Furthermore, competition for resources can leave issues important to disadvantaged groups without adequate support because they often do not get the same attention as those that are important to other, more advantaged groups.

These shortcomings have roots in the cancer control system itself. Thus, ultimately, addressing these issues will fundamentally require a complex systems engineering approach, a fact that has been the guiding theme of this report. Such an approach, even though well appreciated in concept, could be largely uncharted territory for those currently involved in the front lines of various cancer control activities. There are, however, other areas where such a systems approach is already in effect, and it will be possible to learn from the successes and failures in these areas in working to design a systems approach to improving cancer control for broad benefit.

CONCLUSIONS

It is not a new observation that integrated efforts are more effective than uncoordinated ones or that systematic efforts have a greater chance of success than those that are lacking important components. Nonetheless, because of its history, the nation's cancer control system currently fails to follow an integrated systems perspective, and any substantive evaluation of what is required to materially and accountably improve cancer control in the United States would need to start with this acknowledgment. Thus,

Conclusion 1: Cancer control efforts in the United States have generally been cognizant of the need for integrated and accountable approaches across policies and programmatic operations. This notion has long existed in intent but not in practice.

Conclusion 2: The current divergences in cancer control practices could have adverse impacts on the population health and the global economic standing of the United States. The pursuit of numerous uncoordinated efforts fueled by a variety of missions, rationales, incentives, and interests in the public, private, and other sectors has created a situation in which no clear view of the state and the performance of the cancer control system exists.

Conclusion 3: Practicing cancer control solely as prevention or treatment or cure or palliative care or survivorship services, as has been influenced by the historical patterns of funding and specialization, does not allow for comprehensive systems analyses of trade-offs and investments. These realities have impeded the realization of a cancer control system that can robustly drive down the cumulative costs, disparities, and other burdens imposed by cancers.

Conclusion 4: Complexities and divergences in the practice of cancer control also contribute to the complexities in assessing the costs associated with cancer control efforts. Improved financial accounting and accountability are vital prerequisites and ongoing requirements for making informed decisions in a national cancer control strategy.

Conclusion 5: Cancer control has typically been pursued as a "war," "conquest," or "moon shot," but instead it needs to be recognized and approached in practice as a complex adaptive system whose elements are interactive and influential at multiple levels of society, starting with the individual. This change in mind-set is essential to recognize, reduce, and mitigate risks and make significant progress in diminishing the cancer burden in the United States, a situation challenged by population aging and other demographic factors with no apparent blunting of costs across cancer control activities.

As the goals and performances of the cancer control system in the United States have variably evolved, so have the resulting outcomes that particularly affect disadvantaged populations.

Conclusion 6: The performance of the cancer control system as currently constituted in the United States is nowhere near the best-case scenario in the sense of generating effective outcomes, particularly for vulnerable and disadvantaged individuals. Indeed, the current cancer control system is ill equipped to analyze and address the prevailing disparities across all populations resulting from the economic and other incentives and disincentives in place. The remedy for this requires strong policy action.

Taking actions to guide the innately complex adaptive nature of the cancer control system will first require assembling a sophisticated picture of the entire system, its components, and their interactions in constantly changing environments and from multiple viewpoints and necessarily requiring leadership from the federal government.

Conclusion 7: Experiences gained in the realm of urban planning, national security, aviation, financial services, global supply chain logistics, and flood and infection control programs, among other social priority areas, show expanding appreciation and effective applications of systems engineering techniques. The contrast with cancer control lies in the pragmatic reality that these other sectors have long recognized the need to adopt principles of complex adaptive systems to better understand and respond to multiple constituencies, demands, and time scales.

Conclusion 8: The current processes and systems of cancer control are at best reactive to circumstances. A proactive and progressive planning system for cancer control policies and operations would necessitate a learning mind-set, from individuals to institutions, focused on periodically determining what activities should be initiated, expanded, or terminated, as well as critically analyzing the trade-offs and tracking the consequences of related decisions.

Conclusion 9: Cancer control policies have historically and prominently involved directives from the U.S. Congress or the executive branch. Implementing a national cancer control plan involving multiple federal agencies would need congressional or executive branch action to direct operational and resource integration among the participants and to ensure the agencies do not continue to operate in isolation pursuing their own interests.

Conclusion 10: The design of a single top-down, static blueprint for cancer control programs and operations in the United States is currently neither realistic nor productive. Instead, greater effectiveness in cancer control requires centrally available customizable planning tools that are useful across contexts and that can actively support performance monitoring and accountability reviews. Dynamic data feeds, computational and other capabilities, and interactive visual analytics will be required to provide capabilities to enable the supporting systems analyses.

These conclusions form the basis for the following recommendations.

RECOMMENDATIONS

The committee was charged with developing a national strategy for cancer control. Thus, the recommendations below define the key principles, attributes, methods, and tools needed to achieve the goal of implementing an effective national cancer control plan. It is beyond the scope of this report to lay forth the exact details of a plan—in the spirit of a recipe book—or customize a plan and supply numerical targets for multiple stakeholders according to their interests. Even if this exercise was actually possible within the scope of this study, and the lists were included as part of this report to monitor and guide the national cancer control system in desired directions over specific time ranges, it is very likely that those specifics may not be accepted across the variety of stakeholder groups. Convergent decisions require a convergence in goals across many participants, and these are best thought through and settled in a cooperative format—the main argument of this report. The following recommendations therefore will inherently require joint action and resources with the support of a systems monitoring and planning tool to track the state of cancer control efforts and the resulting changes in health.

While a multi-agency approach may necessarily take some time to come to fruition or may not be seen as a possibility depending on the political circumstances, such an effort would be central to ultimately make significant progress in achieving national goals for cancer control. Coming up with a list of action items for each participant or sponsor—with variable criteria—would have been counterproductive both for this report and the national strategic vision based on a complex adaptive systems engineering approach. Moreover, developing a monitoring and planning tool to support the national strategy will require a major project by a group of stakeholders from across the cancer control system with varied competencies and purviews. No one agency, not even the Department of Health and Human Services (HHS) or major tech companies, would have all the capabilities that will be necessary to design and provide support for a prototype. Therefore, it is vital to involve as many entities with a stake and resources in cancer control in formulation of an adaptive national plan.

RECOMMENDATION A: A U.S. National Cancer Control Plan should principally ensure resource integration and operational coordination across the various components of the cancer control system, and should actively do the following:

1. **Improve, where feasible, effective, and affordable, the availability of preventive, screening, diagnostic, and therapeutic interventions. Encourage timely palliative care, hospice care, survivorship services, and related social services according to the preferences and values of patients and their families.**

2. Leverage the advances in and apply "multi-omic" diagnostics to improve therapies and better understand their scientific, clinical, and economic impacts, including their role in creating additional new prospects for cancer control and overall cost reduction.
3. Integrate the use of social, behavioral, and other information made possible by the convergence of communication, social media, cognitive, financial, and sensor technologies as well as electronic health records, cancer registries, and insurance claims to establish large-scale interoperable data sources.
4. Use cloud computing, machine learning, and artificial intelligence tools for continuous analytics, rapid reporting of trends and patterns, and improved forecasting and performance reviews. Evaluate emerging data-intensive technologies not only for their utility in advancing health and economic parameters but also regarding their ability to protect individual privacy and the security of data systems.
5. Apply the tools of complex systems analyses for assessing the "value" of cancer control interventions, establishing robust policy and incentive assessments to guide the development and commercialization of products and services, developing new financing and payment mechanisms that alleviate overall cost burden, and aiding individual patients and their families in making informed decisions about cancer care.
6. Minimize the waste and harm stemming from disparate clinical practices, interventions lacking evidence of effectiveness, and conflicting clinical practice guidelines.
7. Track and monitor financial links, incentives, and disincentives throughout the processes and systems of cancer control and rigorously require conflict-of-interest disclosures across cancer care, research, and patient advocacy activities.
8. Expand and support reproducibility strategies for developing reliable evidence in cancer control from biomedical, clinical, public health, and social science research.
9. Discourage direct-to-consumer marketing and advertising of clinical products and services from companies, medical centers, intermediary firms, and other organizations by terminating the tax deductibility of these business expenses. Furthermore, tighten and enforce rules to particularly curb promotional tactics and strategies that are likely to mislead patients about the benefits of products and care services not based on strong evidence.

10. **Launch and expand public engagement, literacy, and outreach activities, starting with K–12 curriculums and through technology platforms, to broaden the understanding of cancer prevention as an integral component of a healthy life course.**

The history of cancer control efforts in the United States prominently features the involvement of the U.S. Congress or the executive branch in launching new or expanded national initiatives. Coordinating a wide range of federal agencies active in cancer control efforts could require congressional action if the participating agencies lack a legislative authority, in which case it is urged that the U.S. Congress provide the direction to implement the following recommendations.

RECOMMENDATION B: A U.S. National Cancer Control Plan should be led by the Department of Health and Human Services in cooperation with the Office of Management and Budget, Department of Education, Environmental Protection Agency, Department of Defense, Department of Veterans Affairs, Department of Housing and Urban Development, Department of Agriculture, Social Security Administration, Department of Labor, Department of Commerce, Office of Personnel Management, Equal Employment Opportunity Commission, and Department of the Treasury. The Government Accountability Office should periodically review and report to the relevant congressional committees about the achievement of goals specified in the plan.

A national cancer control plan will need to include all these federal participants, in particular, in undertaking a comprehensive review of diverse and shifting needs and an integration of available resources and capabilities, with accountability for periodic performance review and reporting annually, with a rigorous review every 3–4 years, similar to the congressionally mandated assessments in other area. While this extensive level of cooperation and collaboration among multiple government agencies and parties may seem daunting, there are precedents for such an approach. The U.S. Global Change Research Program, for instance, involves 13 federal agencies that jointly produce the quadrennial *National Climate Assessment*. The most recent report in 2018 was produced by a team of more than 300 experts guided by a 60-member Federal Advisory Committee, and it was then extensively reviewed by the public and experts, including federal agencies and a panel of the National Academy of Sciences.[1] Similarly, the National HIV/AIDS Strategy involves the Department of Homeland Security, Department of Defense (DoD), Department of the Interior, Department of Justice, Department of Labor, Department of Education, Equal Employment Opportunity Commission, HHS, Department of Housing and Urban Development, Social Security Administration, Department of State, and Department of Veterans Affairs.

Another example is the NextGen air control system, discussed in Chapter 3, which requires integrative work and ongoing coordination and diligent performance review across many different agencies, particularly involving industrial partnership. And, indeed, the original Apollo "moon shot" that has inspired much of the recent activities in cancer control was a working demonstration of synergy among more than 20 different government agencies operating under a congressional mandate. Other prominent examples include the expectation from the U.S. Congress that 16 U.S. government agencies, comprising DoD and the intelligence sector, work together on national security issues. Similarly, the recommendations from the bipartisan Blue Ribbon Study Panel on Biodefense, which led to the 2018 National Biodefense Strategy from the White House, mandates HHS to implement multi-agency projects.

Moreover, the ultimate success or failure of the national cancer plan will depend on gaining a functional understanding of the nation's cancer control system and being able to predict how it responds to various interests and pressures. Therefore,

RECOMMENDATION C: In support of the U.S. National Cancer Control Plan, the Department of Health and Human Services and the federal partner agencies should fund and support an independent organization—or a consortium—with principal competencies in systems engineering, industrial design, software development, and information and visual analytics to prototype and develop a publicly available, interactive, and evolvable planning and monitoring tool.

Moreover,
C-1: Periodic consultations with key participants from state and local governments and for-profit and nonprofit sectors should focus on ensuring that data feeds to the planning tool are customized and

[1] U.S. Global Change Research Program. 2018. *Impacts, Risks, and Adaptation in the United States: Fourth National Climate Assessment*, Volume II [Reidmiller, D. R., C. W. Avery, D. R. Easterling, K. E. Kunkel, K. L. M. Lewis, T. K. Maycock, and B. C. Stewart (eds.)]. U.S. Global Change Research Program, Washington, DC.

routinely refreshed and that planning parameters are properly applied and extensively tested for transparency and meaningfulness.
C-2: Leaders from multiple sectors—biomedical, consumer products and services, computing, information technology, financial, transportation, agricultural, and construction—should be engaged through an advisory council mechanism.

It would be counterproductive and economically unfeasible if the various stakeholders each went about developing its own platform; hence the need for a "master version." An exemplar can be found in the weather forecasting systems of the National Oceanic and Atmospheric Administration; the agency also relies on its own scientific programs and numerous groups like Google, NASA, and local TV stations for disseminating the information broadly. The development of the planning and monitoring tool will need to be overseen by a group of individuals with knowledge and competence in a large variety of areas in business and society (the Federal Aviation Administration's NextGen Advisory Committee could serve as an initial exemplar for the advisory procedures). The tool will also require as much up-to-date data about the nation's cancer system as possible, so it will be important, for instance, that each state and territory bring and upload its own data sets—and refresh them periodically on a cloud-based repository for comparisons and meta-reports as well as custom analyses. Large-scale tools such as this one envisioned for cancer control can be seen in regular use elsewhere in applications for monitoring, for example, the economy, financial markets, labor dynamics, classified intelligence, and the manufacturing supply chain.

APPLYING THE GUIDANCE SYSTEM

Assuming that agreement has been reached that developing a guidance system for the existing cancer control system is a worthwhile goal, how might such a guidance system work? The precise details—and even many of the broad characteristics—of such a system will depend on exactly what it is intended to do, but here is one potential approach relating to the planning and monitoring tool.

The possible outputs of the planning and monitoring tool(s) would necessarily include all the cancer-related variables that might be of value to policy makers, including cancer incidence rates and mortality rates, quality-of-life indicators or proxies, the cost of a policy and its effects on the nation's gross domestic product, workforce productivity gains, and so on. It will be crucial that the inputs to the simulation package of the tool include the various policy actions that are possible to guide the cancer control system, from spending levels on various research and prevention efforts to policies concerning health insurance (including Medicare and Medicaid), public health campaigns, policies on drug patents and pricing, and environmental carcinogens. The goal of such a tool should be to allow policy makers to get answers to questions of the form "How will instituting policies A, B, and C affect outputs X, Y, and Z?" The linked simulations and visualizations of the tool would make it possible to generate real-time dashboards to compare different approaches to cancer control. With this information in hand, it will be up to decision makers in different areas to compare and decide on which policies to pursue.

Such a suite of simulations could be used in various ways. Suppose, for example, that federal policy makers wished to compare the benefits, broadly defined, of treatment or prevention. The visuals could predict what range of outcomes are possible through treatments (such as immunotherapies) versus public health campaigns to mitigate disease risks (e.g., campaigns to encourage people to get human papillomavirus vaccines) and could also include the effects of various possible non-fiscal government policies (e.g., changes to patent regulations or tax and housing policies). An advantage of the sort of multi-criteria systems analysis described in Chapter 3 is that it could take into account many different factors of interest to stakeholders.

Another potential use could be to look for the policies that would have the greatest effect on reducing disparities in cancer burden. With a simulated output that included details about various cancer-related differences among socioeconomic groups, such as behavioral differences (alcohol consumption, as an instance), differences in health insurance coverage, differences in treatments and their adherence, and also details about what sorts of factors affect those differences (as in education, outreach, and social security), it should be possible to examine how well various policies would serve to reduce inequities. Through this kind of systems analysis, policy makers could derive a package of policies with the best chance of closing the gaps in cancer outcomes among various groups.

The ultimate success of this approach will depend mainly on two factors: the quality of the modeling and simulations and how closely policy makers adhere to the indicated plans. It is difficult at this point to predict just how well a simulation of the cancer control system will be able to forecast the behavior of the real system. The tool and its constituent models would be far more ambitious than any simulation that has yet been built for cancer control. But what seems clear is that even a less than perfect simulation should lead people to think more deeply and clearly about how the different components of the cancer control system interact and should give valuable insights into the system's behavior and how to modify it. That in itself could make the effort to develop the planning and monitoring tool worthwhile, and ultimately, with enough design improvements and testing, it should be feasible to simulate the cancer control system that represents and predicts its behavior with reasonable accuracy.

FROM MANY TO ONE: ADVANCING THE PRACTICE

As noted earlier, this report does not include lists of customized actions that stakeholders can take instantly to improve cancer control—for example, that agency X should be doing more of this or less of that, to what extent, when, and for how long. This is a direct consequence of the committee charge as well as the report's findings that the current approaches to cancer control are collectively not performing to their best and should be replaced with a systems-oriented approach. Near- or short-term recommendations would simply be more of the same—actions intended to improve one aspect of the overall system without a clear understanding of how those actions would play out in the context of the entire cancer control system.

Indeed, from the committee's point of view, offering such short-term recommendations could actually be counterproductive because it would buttress today's common belief that the appropriate way to improve cancer control is to seek to improve the individual components of the system in isolation—and would thus undercut the main message of this report.

Given this situation, then, what should the various cancer control actors be doing until an overarching approach can be developed that addresses cancer control with systems engineering? The stakeholders can begin shaping their actions with an eye toward how those actions fit within the broader cancer control system, with emphasis on the core principles laid out in recommendation A. To illustrate the sorts of things that this might entail, consider the following suggestions.

Disease Control and Prevention

The Centers for Disease Control and Prevention (CDC), as a leader in disease control and prevention, has sponsored a variety of cancer-related programs with a wide range of objectives and is one of the major governmental agencies in U.S. efforts to control cancer. It supports research on a number of cancer-related topics, including studies on cancer incidence and mortality, examinations of the effectiveness of various cancer control efforts, and studies of public knowledge and attitudes about different types of cancer. Its National Program of Cancer Registries supports the collection of data by state cancer registries across the United States and takes part in publishing those data. It sponsors a number of relevant programs such as the National Comprehensive Cancer Control Program, the National Breast and Cervical Cancer Early Detection Program, the National Program of Cancer Registries, and the Colorectal Cancer Control Program.[2] Its National Institute for Occupational Safety and Health conducts research and makes recommendations on workplace exposures to cancer-causing chemicals. And its Office on Smoking and Health carries out a number of activities intended to reduce smoking-related disease, particularly lung cancer. These activities include programs that seek to keep young people from starting smoking, the promotion of smoke-free environments, programs that help people who smoke to quit, and actions designed to reduce smoking-related health disparities among various groups.

There are a number of changes or additions that CDC could make to this suite of programs in anticipation of a future in which a more systems-oriented approach is taken to cancer control. For example, the agency could develop rigorous ways to compare the effectiveness of its different programs across different contexts. It would still be necessary to make judgments about the composite value of various outcomes—as in tobacco cessation and prevention interventions—and how those outcomes affect a larger, interconnected system of cancer control. This could involve joint analyses of efforts between CDC and its sister agencies within HHS. Such studies of the interactions among various segments of the cancer control system could provide insights and knowledge that would be valuable in developing an accurate model of the entire system.

Among the many CDC programs, perhaps the closest in spirit to the vision described in this report is its National Comprehensive Cancer Control Program (NCCCP), established in 1998. It funds and provides guidance and technical assistance to states, territories, and other entities for developing their individual comprehensive cancer control plans. NCCCP emphasizes a multi-pronged approach to cancer control, with a focus on primary prevention, early detection and treatment, and supporting cancer survivors and caregivers, and it supports these focus areas through what it terms "cross-cutting priorities." These priorities include supporting changes in policies, systems, and environments to make communities healthier;[3] achieving health equity; and using evaluations to assess and demonstrate outcomes, and these priorities can be multi-pronged in nature as well. The priority of building healthy communities, for example, emphasizes the development of policies to protect people from harmful exposures (such as to secondhand smoke), the creation of systems that influence people to make healthier choices (such as eating better or getting screened for cancer), and changes in the local environment to

[2] This text has been revised since prepublication release.
[3] This text has been revised since prepublication release.

encourage individuals to be more active (such as adding bike lanes or walking paths).

These plans explicitly recognize the importance of addressing cancer control on multiple fronts at once, but in general they do not take the next step and approach cancer control as a complex adaptive system. Instead, the plans typically take an isolated, one-item-at-a-time approach: to accomplish A, do B; to accomplish C, do D; and so on. In particular, they do not take into account the way different components of the cancer control system can interact and affect one another. Furthermore, while the plans may set priorities, there is generally no way to objectively compare the performance of different combinations of strategies in order to zero in on an overall strategy that will be most effective.

Because of the plans' explicit acknowledgment of the importance of a comprehensive approach to cancer control, NCCCP would be an excellent program to enhance through a systems engineering approach to cancer control while a national plan is being developed with numerous participants. CDC could, for example, test a prototype of the interactive planning and monitoring tool described in recommendation C by making it available to the states and other entities for use in developing their comprehensive plans. Such a tool could be less complex and less layered because it may not include various options at the national level, such as federal funding for cancer research or national policies that affect medical care, drug prices or advanced technologies. Still, even this simplified version of the planning and monitoring tool would make it possible to get feedback from dozens of different organizations concerning what worked well—feedback that could be used in the development of the national tool.

Biomedical and Clinical Research

The National Cancer Institute (NCI) has been responsible for a large percentage of cancer research funding in the United States. The basic research supported by NCI, in particular, has motivated much of the progress in treating cancer over the past several decades. The basic cancer biology program is complemented by a population sciences program that studies cancer incidence and progression using epidemiology, genetics, and behavioral and social sciences to understand and predict risk and also to improve the quality of life for cancer survivors. Insights from this population research have been applied in studies that seek to find the most effective cancer prevention methods. Yet another line of research is focused on the clinical diagnosis and treatment of cancer, with a major goal being the development, improvement, and comparison of therapeutic interventions to improve patient outcomes.

In addition to these major areas of research, which are the responsibility of a half dozen NCI divisions, the institute has a number of centers focused on specific topics. The goal of the Center for Cancer Genomics, for instance, is to unify the various cancer genomics research activities that take place across NCI, while the Center to Reduce Cancer Health Disparities seeks to find ways to reduce inequities in cancer incidence, treatment, and outcomes. The Center for Research Strategy takes a higher-level view of NCI research, looking for research gaps and opportunities. The Center for Strategic Scientific Initiatives, which is focused on cutting-edge approaches and technologies, explores new scientific discoveries and emerging technologies with the goal of developing novel preventive agents, diagnostics, and therapies.

Given the broad range of research that takes place under the auspices of NCI, the agency has a tremendous opportunity to synthesize the knowledge and insights that will be necessary for the systems approach to cancer control envisioned in this report. For example, the interactive planning and monitoring tool described in recommendation C will be effective only to the degree that it is possible to predict the outcomes of various possible strategies with some reliability—and, in particular, to have some information about how the outcomes of different strategies compare. Thus, one valuable service that NCI can provide would be to also carry out rigorous comparisons of effectiveness across interventions, looking at the outcomes of different approaches in varying circumstances—including conducting financial analyses of research dollars spent on prevention strategies versus treatment, for instance, or of research funding for developing novel pharmaceuticals versus improved techniques for early detection and establishing robust reproducibility standards for research supported or conducted by NCI as well as different units of NIH involved in cancer research. One goal of the proposed tool is to allow policy makers to compare the likely outcomes of different strategies, but the tool will be only as good as the data informing it.

A second opportunity for NCI would be to move further beyond the usual specialties and deliberately advance research that examines intersectional issues. How, for example, do new developments in cancer control affect the behavior of clinicians or of patients? It is well known, for instance, that improvements in auto safety led to an increase in risky driving, as drivers believed the safer cars allowed them to take more chances. Could something similar happen in the cancer field? Would improved treatment of melanoma lead some individuals to be more willing to risk significant sun exposure, or would an effective treatment for lung cancer lead to an increase in the number of smokers? There are many ways in which the different components of the cancer control system interact with and affect one another, and these could be valuable subjects for study.

Advocacy and Outreach

Among the numerous nonprofit organizations involved in advocacy and outreach for cancer control, some of them, such as the American Cancer Society, are generalists and concern themselves with all aspects of cancer control, from basic research to helping cancer survivors, but most are specialized in one way or another. Most types of cancer—lung cancer, breast cancer, ovarian cancer, prostate cancer, colon cancer, leukemia and lymphoma, and so on—have at least one nonprofit devoted to them, and different aspects of cancer control, such as survivorship care, are also represented. Most of these nonprofits advocate with policy makers for their particular, sometimes narrow, interests. Many of them support research in hopes of improving prevention or detection or treatment, while others are devoted to helping cancer patients and their families in various ways.

Similarly, there are professional organizations devoted to practically every aspect of cancer control, with a focus on individual types of cancer, different types of treatments, or different phases in the cancer control continuum. Many organizations have been created to represent professionals working on different aspects of cancer control, including physicians, nurses, social workers, and patient navigators as well as informal caregivers. While these organizations clearly portray the immense variety of common and potentially competing interests, they also offer opportunities to connect directly with the many different professionals who populate the cancer control network.

Individually, each of these organizations touches on only a small portion of the entire cancer control system, but collectively they cover most, if not all, of it. Thus, one way these organizations could help move cancer control forward toward the future strategic vision of this report would be to make stronger connections among themselves and help the system become more integrated. The first step would be simply to encourage a greater awareness of the entire cancer control system and its nature, with individual components interacting to achieve the overarching goals, and the necessity for a planning and monitoring tool to organize and integrate the planning efforts necessary for national cancer control. Then organizations could develop connections among themselves that followed the lines of mutual interests or approaches. This could have immediate payoffs—if, say, two or more organizations pooled their resources to accomplish ends that were important to all of them—but the more important return will be found in the long term, as these interconnections help build a much more integrated cancer control system in which a systems approach is much more likely to be effective.

BUILDING NEW CAPABILITIES AND COMPETENCIES

Today's cancer control system is populated by highly trained and dedicated professionals. They have developed exactly the sorts of capabilities and competencies that have been asked of them and then put those skills to work in the system as they found it. As discussed, however, the current system has more than a few inefficiencies and weaknesses that could amplify the burden on society. A complex adaptive systems approach to cancer control will require a new set of capabilities and competencies not only in the analysts and policy makers who concern themselves with the performance of the entire system but also in many of those working to prevent, detect, and treat, cancers, and caring for survivors as well as those approaching death.

At the present time, most of those in the various cancer control communities—from oncologists to biomedical researchers in laboratories across universities and companies, and from public health practitioners to those involved in palliative care and end-of-life care—are focused mainly on their own specialties. They may communicate and cooperate with those in other areas when necessary, but most of the time, that is not the case. That is the state of the current system.

Moving toward a more systemic and systematic approach to cancer control will require understanding and performing one's job in a much broader context. It will require communication with a much broader range of participants than is common now, for instance, and also the ability to understand and appreciate the goals and concerns of those working in other areas. It will require a degree of awareness of the state and performance of the overall system and a sense of one's place within that system. This sort of systems awareness has been fruitfully achieved in various other systems, from the National Airspace System to just-in-time automobile manufacturing system, although none is as large and diverse as the cancer control system. Part of building that systems awareness will be developing the capabilities and competencies—with corresponding implications for education, research practices, and professional incentives—necessary to engage with and guide a complex adaptive system.

More than anything, what will be required will be the development of a systems mind-set, which involves seeing the world and one's position in it in terms of the systems one is working in. Not everyone may embrace this broad mind-set in practice, but it will be required of decision makers, and it will be helpful to most participants so that they can understand how they fit into the big picture. People with this mind-set see themselves as part of a large effort with many parts, much like air traffic controllers in the National Airspace System, for example. They know how to do their jobs—directing planes in their airspace—but they also have an understanding of how their work can affect others in different parts of the system—and how others or the weather can affect them.

The development of this mind-set and the requisite competencies and capabilities will not happen overnight. Two key steps will advance this process. The first is the development and dissemination of the cancer control planning and monitoring tool. Those who learn about how the tool is used—and, ideally, get the chance to work with the tool themselves, at least to a limited degree—will naturally begin to think of the nation's cancer control efforts as all part of one large, sprawling, loosely connected system. The second step will be in bringing together those from various specialties and divisions of cancer control—and, importantly, beyond—to develop shared implementation plans, which hopefully would be in line with the overall direction decided on based on the tool's projections. This sort of communication and collaboration is a precondition to developing any shared responsibility or strategy for the entire cancer control system.

WORKING FOR SUCCESS

For patients, the fragmentation of today's system is perhaps its most negative feature. Divided practices force patients to play a major role in the coordination of their own care, making sure that the proper information is communicated from one part of the system to another, and they are the ones who bear the consequences when communication between the different components of the system breaks down (for instance, a situation that leaves a patient's oncologist uninformed about a condition of which the patient's primary clinician is well aware). Thus, to many patients, the main sign that improvements in the cancer control system have occurred might be better integration of the system, with the separate pieces working together seamlessly. The current or envisioned system of cancer control may never be able to be fully integrated; however, it might be enough for it to be coordinated well enough that the patient is never aware of the gaps between the pieces.

For policy makers focused on cancer care, the success of the system will be most defined by how well various goals are met, such as lowering cancer incidence and death rates, improving certain health status indicators after a cancer diagnosis, and reducing costs while maintaining quality. For others, policies pertaining to the environment, housing, tax, social security, defense, and veterans could provide adjacent insights for cancer control. These kinds of composite understandings in turn will depend on the accuracy of the model's forecasts, so success will also require a model that reliably and accurately simulates the main aspects of the cancer control system and predicts the outcomes of various policy measures.

Success will also depend on how well this systems approach engages, rather than alienates, the frontline participants in cancer control in carrying out the simulation-informed plan. It is worth noting that the modeling could actually forecast how well various changes would be accepted by participants, particularly using established and emerging insights from social and behavioral sciences, and could even simulate different ways of instituting those changes to determine which approaches would likely be most successful.

Over time, though, success will be defined by how well the cancer control system succeeds in achieving two prime qualities: accountability and equity. One of the advantages of the type of planning and monitoring tool that has been discussed here is that it encourages a decision process that is open and accountable. As was the case with the multi-criteria systems analytic approaches described in Chapter 3, a cancer control model and simulation of the sort under discussion would produce rankings of various options according to explicit inclusion and weightings of various factors. There can be disagreement and debate about how the different factors should be weighted, depending on the participants in the discussion—how, for example, should a case of cancer prevented be valued versus a case of cancer cured or brought into remission versus how should a drug be priced for a particular kind of cancer?—but the model itself would make clear exactly what choices are being made. Once those choices have been made, the model identifies the path most likely to produce the best outcome according to the available information and user-provided weights. Regular monitoring of the system with changing data sets will determine whether the real outcomes match the predicted outcomes.

In a way, the use of the tool could encourage greater openness and accountability by the way it is operated. People can debate the choices, but once a decision has been made, the path is determined, and accountability becomes mainly a matter of making sure that the various components of the cancer control system are performing as expected and progress is being made, measured, and reported. If the outcome differs significantly from what was predicted, that would quickly become apparent because of the regular monitoring of the system, and modifications could be made—all done openly and with accountability.

Similarly, the use of a planning and monitoring tool of the type under discussion here offers perhaps our best chance of lessening the degree of inequity in cancer care in the United States. The inequity in the system today is the product of a number of interacting factors—social inequalities, financial inequalities, educational inequalities, behavioral differences, disparities in medical care, and so forth. In other words, the inequities are a systems issue rather than being the product of one or a few factors that can be addressed independently. Inequities might even be an emergent property of these systemic interactions. Thus, complex systems analyses will be a prerequisite to address disparities in cancer control, where a number of different factors are recognized, analyzed, and addressed simultaneously. There is no way to do this with today's cancer control system; a complex systems engineering approach guided by a multi-level, multi-criteria model of the cancer control system could be an effective way to make progress.

SETTING A PRECEDENT

National cancer control efforts require something unprecedented: a collaborative initiative among multiple participants to develop a joint ability with joint accountability to understand and guide in productive ways a complex adaptive system. The interactive planning and monitoring tool required for this work will demand both the development of new capabilities and the repurposing of existing resources that could be fruitfully integrated into a functional system. Such a system would not only be invaluable in cancer control but could also be useful in many other areas where complex adaptive systems are involved—practically every aspect of population health. The stakes are extremely high. Projections indicate that the number of cancer cases will overwhelm the current health and medical system capacity as early as the next decade. The nation's cancer control system will need to become much more effective, efficient, and accountable than it is today—indeed, it will require a major transformation to successfully address the approaching wave of cancers. Guiding the cancer control system using the science and engineering of complex adaptive systems offers productive possibilities for progress, including effectively integrating and coordinating the resources and intentions of groups and individuals.

Appendix A

Stakeholder Input

A public workshop titled How to Transform Cancer Control was organized in June 2018. One-half of that workshop was focused on "What have we learned in the past decade?" and included the following discussion questions: "What major insights, developments, and barriers have led to the current realities of understanding, practice, and policies across the cancer control continuum?" and, "How can policies and programmatic efforts that have not met their stated aspirations and goals for cancer control inform and guide our next steps?" The second half of the workshop was centered on what should be done differently, and the focus questions were: "What strategic capabilities could maximize the scientific, technologic, clinical, field level, regulatory, and financial results, and their unified impact on cancer control?" and, "The current mismatches in goals and implementation as well as with the supporting information (technologics) across different stakeholder groups hinder progress throughout the cancer control continuum. What should be done differently?"

The following stakeholders provided input and participated in discussions, along with other members of the public who also attended the workshop.

ANNA BARKER, Arizona State University
OTIS BRAWLEY, American Cancer Society
JULIA BRODY, Silent Spring Institute
DAVID CHAMBERS, National Cancer Institute

CHRISTOPHER COGLE, University of Florida
ERIC FEUER, National Cancer Institute
LESLIE GIVEN, Strategic Health Concepts
GEORGE HRIPCSAK, Columbia University and New York–Presbyterian Hospital
DENNIS McBRIDE, Source America
CHARLES PHELPS, University of Rochester
ELIZABETH PLATZ, Johns Hopkins Bloomberg School of Public Health
HOLLY PRIGERSON, Weill Cornell Medicine
LISA RICHARDSON, Centers for Disease Control and Prevention
LOUISE RUSSELL, University of Pennsylvania
JAY SCHNITZER, MITRE Corporation
LEE SCHWARTZBERG, West Cancer Center

Appendix B

Biographical Information

Michael M. E. Johns, M.D. (*Chair*), is the chancellor emeritus and a professor of medicine and public health at Emory University. He was previously the executive vice president for health affairs and president, chief executive officer, and chair of Emory Healthcare. He has also served as interim executive vice president for medical affairs at the University of Michigan and vice president of the medical faculty and dean of the Johns Hopkins School of Medicine and has been on the faculty of the University of Virginia and the Walter Reed Army Medical Center. He is a member of the board of the Uniformed Services University of the Health Sciences, the Vanderbilt University Medical Center, and the University of Michigan Health. He has also served on the advisory committee to the director of the Centers for Disease Control and Prevention, as editor of the *Archives of Otolaryngology*, and on the editorial board of the *Journal of the American Medical Association*. He received his bachelor's degree at Wayne State University and graduated with a medical degree with distinction from the University of Michigan, where he also completed his residency training in otolaryngology, head, and neck surgery. He is the former president of the American Board of Otolaryngology. He has served on various boards, including those of AMN Healthcare, Blue Cross and Blue Shield of Maryland, Georgia Cancer Coalition, Johnson & Johnson, and West Health. His numerous honors include the Castle Connolly Lifetime Achievement Award and an honorary doctorate of science from the University of Michigan. He is a member and former vice chair of the council of the National Academy of Medicine.

Katrina Armstrong, M.D., is the Jackson Professor of Clinical Medicine at the Harvard Medical School and the chair of the Department of Medicine and physician-in-chief of Massachusetts General Hospital. Previously she was the chief of the Division of General Internal Medicine, an associate director of the Abramson Cancer Center, and a co-director of the Robert Wood Johnson Clinical Scholars Program at the University of Pennsylvania. She has been a fellow at the Leonard Davis Institute of Health Economics and a senior scholar at the Center for Clinical Epidemiology and Biostatistics at the University of Pennsylvania. She is the chair of the external advisory panel of the Clinical Sequencing Exploratory Research Consortium of the National Human Genome Research Institute. Her honors include the Molly and Sidney N. Zubrow Award and the Robert Austrian Faculty Award from the University of Pennsylvania School of Medicine, the Warfield T. Longcope Prize for Excellence in Clinical Medicine from the Johns Hopkins University School of Medicine, and a Robert Wood Johnson Faculty Scholar Award. She is a graduate of Yale University and the Johns Hopkins University School of Medicine. She is a fellow of the American College of Physicians, a member of the American Society of Clinical Investigation, and a member of the National Academy of Medicine.

Smita Bhatia, M.D., M.P.H., is the Gay and Bew White Endowed Chair in Pediatric Oncology at the University of Alabama School of Medicine, where she is also the director of the Institute for Cancer Outcomes and Survivorship at the University of Alabama School of Medicine. She is also the associate director for outcomes research at the University of Alabama Comprehensive Cancer Center. She has served on the editorial board of the *Journal of Clinical Oncology*. She obtained her M.B.B.S. and M.D. from the All India Institute of Medical Sciences, where she also completed her internship and residency. She received an M.P.H. from the University of Minnesota and completed her fellowship in blood banking, pediatric hematology/oncology, and bone marrow transplantation. She has served on the board of the American Society of Clinical Oncology. She is an elected member of the Association of American Physicians, the American Pediatric Society, and the American Society for Clinical Investigation.

Betty Ferrell, R.N., Ph.D., is a director and a professor at the City of Hope National Medical Center, where she directs the Division of Nursing Research and Education. She has been the co-chair of the National Consensus Project for Quality Palliative Care led by the National Coalition for Hospice and Palliative Care. She is a co-editor of the *Oxford Textbook of Palliative Nursing* and the editor-in-chief of the *Journal of Hospice & Palliative Nursing*. She received a B.S.N. from Central State University, a

Ph.D. from Texas Woman's University, and an M.A. in theology, ethics, and culture from Claremont Graduate University. She is a recipient of the American Cancer Society Pathfinder Award and was named one of the 30 visionaries in the field of hospice and palliative medicine by the American Academy of Hospice and Palliative Medicine. She has been a member of the board of scientific advisors of the National Cancer Institute and the National Cancer Policy Forum of the National Academies of Sciences, Engineering, and Medicine. She is a fellow of the American Psychosocial Oncology Society, American Academy of Nursing, and Palliative Care Nursing.

Jonathan Fielding, M.D., M.P.H., M.B.A., is a distinguished professor of health policy and management and pediatrics in the Fielding School of Public Health and the Geffen School of Medicine at the University of California, Los Angeles (UCLA). He is the founding co-director of the UCLA Center for Health Enhancement, Education, and Research. He was a founding member of the U.S. Preventive Services Task Force and is the chair of the U.S. Community Preventive Services Task Force. He served as the director of public health and a health officer for Los Angeles County for 16 years. Before that he was the Massachusetts Commissioner of Public Health. He has served as the president and a regent for the American College of Preventive Medicine and as a member of the National Commission on Prevention Priorities as well as on the advisory committee to the California State Department of Public Health. His honors include the Sedgwick Medal for Distinguished Service in Public Health, UCLA Medal, Milton and Ruth Roemer Prize for Creative Local Public Health Work, Fries Prize for Improving Health, Porter Prize for National Impact on Improving the Health of Americans, and Beverlee A. Myers Award for Excellence in Public Health, and he received an honorary fellowship from the Society for Public Health Education. He received his M.D., M.A., and M.P.H. from Harvard University and his M.B.A. from the Wharton School of Business Administration. He is a member of the National Academy of Medicine.

Beverly Ashleigh Guadagnolo, M.D., M.P.H., is a professor of radiation oncology and health services research at The University of Texas MD Anderson Cancer Center where she serves as the section chief of sarcoma/melanoma radiation oncology, and she is the associate director of the Physicians Referral Service. She served as member of the Department of Health and Human Services advisory committee on minority health, the Medicare Evidence Development and Advisory Committee of the Centers for Medicare & Medicaid Services, and on a technical expert panel of the Agency for Healthcare Research and Quality project on radiotherapy treatments for head and neck cancer. She received a B.A. in biology from The University of Texas at Austin, an M.D. from the Harvard Medical School, and an M.P.H from the Harvard School of Public Health, where she held a National Cancer Institute fellowship in cancer prevention.

Joseph Lipscomb, Ph.D., is the Georgia Cancer Coalition Distinguished Cancer Scholar and a professor of health policy and management at the Rollins School of Public Health at Emory University. Previously he was the associate director for population sciences at Emory's Winship Cancer Institute and a clinical investigator at the Kaiser Permanente Center for Health Research. He was also on the faculty of Duke University and the University of North Carolina at Chapel Hill, the chief of the Outcomes Research Branch at the National Cancer Institute, and a study director at the National Academies of Sciences, Engineering, and Medicine. He has twice received the National Institutes of Health Award of Merit. He has served as a consultant in health economics, outcomes research, and program evaluation to the American Cancer Society, SRA International, Amgen, Pfizer, Boehringer Ingelheim, Janssen, Dupont Merck, G.D. Searle, the Society of Nuclear Medicine, Burroughs Wellcome, and PhRMA. He is the chair of the Data and Evaluation Committee for the Georgia Cancer Control Consortium and is a member of the American College of Surgeons Commission on Cancer's Quality Integration Committee, and he was the chair of the American Cancer Society Health Services Research Advisory Committee. He received his B.A. from Vanderbilt University and Ph.D. from the University of North Carolina at Chapel Hill.

María Elena Martínez, Ph.D., M.P.H., is the Sam M. Walton Endowed Chair for Cancer Research and a professor of family medicine and public health at the University of California, San Diego. She also serves as the associate director of population sciences, disparities, and community engagement at the Moores Cancer Center. Previously she was a professor of epidemiology in the Mel and Enid Zuckerman College of Public Health and was the Richard H. Hollen Professor of Cancer Prevention at the University of Arizona Cancer Center. She received a B.S. in nutrition from the University of Illinois and an M.P.H. and a Ph.D. in epidemiology from the University of Texas School of Public Health. She completed a postdoctoral fellowship at the Harvard School of Public Health. She is the senior editor of the cancer disparities section for *Cancer Epidemiology, Biomarkers, & Prevention* and an associate editor of the *Journal of the National Cancer Institute*. She has served as the chair of the American Association for Cancer Research's Minorities in Cancer Research Council. She served as a member of the National Cancer Institute's Board of Scientific Advisors and was a member of the Cancer Moonshot Blue Ribbon Panel.

Mary McCabe, R.N., M.A., is a consultant in cancer survivorship. She was formerly the clinical director of the Cancer Survivorship Center and the chair of the ethics committee at the Memorial Sloan Kettering Cancer Center. Previously she served as the director of nursing services at the Lombardi Cancer Center at Georgetown University and as a lecturer at Cornell Weill Medical College and the Columbia University School of Nursing. She has been the director of the Offices of Clinical Research Promotion and of Education and Special Initiatives at the National Cancer Institute, where she was also the assistant director of the Division of Cancer Treatment and Diagnosis. She received her B.A. from Trinity College, B.S.N. from Emory University, and M.A. from The Catholic University of America. Her honors include the American Cancer Society Merit Award, Oncology Nursing Society Leadership Award, National Institutes of Health (NIH) Outstanding Performance Award, NIH Director's Award, and Emory University's Outstanding Alumnae Award.

Leah Merchant is a section supervisor for the Montana Cancer Control Programs in the Montana Department of Public Health and Human Services. Her responsibilities include managing regional contracts with local public health departments across Montana to implement cancer education outreach and direct screening services and also leading statewide implementations efforts to address cancer policy issues affecting diverse populations. She is the past chair of the cancer council of the National Association of Chronic Disease Directors. She received her B.A. degree from Smith College.

Jewel Mullen, M.D., M.P.H., M.P.A., is the associate dean for healthy equity at the Dell Medical School and an associate professor of population health and internal medicine at The University of Texas at Austin. She is the former principal deputy assistant secretary for health, former acting assistant secretary for health, and former acting director of the National Vaccine Program Office at the Department of Health and Human Services. Previously she served as a commissioner of the Connecticut Department of Public Health. Before that she was the director of the Bureau of Community Health and Prevention at the Massachusetts Department of Public Health and the medical director of Baystate Mason Square Neighborhood Health Center. She has served as a member of the advisory committee to the director of the Centers for Disease Control and Prevention and the chair of the Breast and Cervical Cancer Early Detection and Control Advisory Committee. She serves on the editorial board of *Morbidity and Mortality Weekly Report*. She began her clinical career as a member of the National Health Service Corps at Bellevue Hospital, New York, after which she joined the medical faculty of the University of Virginia. She has been a member of the medical staff at the Hospital of St. Raphael, the Yale University Health Services, and Yale New Haven Hospital. She received her B.S. and M.P.H. from Yale University. She received her M.D. from the Icahn School of Medicine at Mount Sinai, completed her internal medicine residency at the University of Pennsylvania, and also received an M.P.A. from Harvard's John F. Kennedy School of Government. She is the former president of the Association of State and Territorial Health Officials.

Electra Paskett, Ph.D., is the Marion N. Rowley Professor of Cancer Research at The Ohio State University. She is also the director of the Division of Cancer Prevention and Control in the College of Medicine, a professor in the Division of Epidemiology, the associate director for population sciences and community outreach at the Comprehensive Cancer Center, and the director of the Center for Cancer Health Equity at The Ohio State University. Previously she was on the faculty of the Wake Forest University School of Medicine. She is a past president of the American Society of Preventive Oncology and was the chair of the American Public Health Association Cancer Forum. She is the deputy editor of *Cancer, Epidemiology, Biomarkers and Prevention* and has served on the editorial boards of *Cancer Prevention Research* and *Cancer*. She received her B.S. from The University of Utah and Ph.D. from the University of Washington. She is a recipient of the American Association for Cancer Research for Outstanding Achievement Award and the American Society of Preventive Oncology Distinguished Achievement Award. She is a fellow of the American Association for the Advancement of Science. She is a member of the National Cancer Advisory Board and has served as the president of the American Society of Preventive Oncology.

George Poste, Ph.D., D.V.M., is a Regent's Professor and the Del E. Webb Chair of Health Innovation and the director and chief scientist of Complex Adaptive Systems at Arizona State University, where he was also the founding director of the Biodesign Institute. Previously he was the chief science and technology officer and president of research and development, among other leadership positions, at SmithKline Beecham (now GlaxoSmithKline). Earlier he was a principal cancer research scientist at Roswell Park Memorial Institute (now Roswell Park Comprehensive Cancer Center). He has served on the Defense Science Board and on boards of numerous companies, including Health Longevity, Inc., Haplogen GmbH, Synthetic Genomics, Caris Life Sciences (as vice-chair), Exelexis, Illumina, Maxygen, diaDexus (as chair; acquired by VaxGen), Structural Genomix (as chair; acquired by Eli Lilly), AdvancePCS (acquired by CVS), Burrill and Company, and Monsanto. He has been a trustee of the Gordon Research Conferences, Royal Society of Medicine Foundation, Institute for Scientific Information, and BP Technology Advisory Council. He has served as a distinguished fellow at the Hoover Institution of Stanford University and on the board of medical governors of the World Economic Forum. He has received honorary doctorates from the University of Bristol (where he received his D.V.M. and Ph.D.) and the University of Dundee. His awards include the Global Business Leadership Forum's Einstein Award and the Pharmaceutical Industry Leadership Forum's Scrip Lifetime Achievement Award. He is a member of the Council on Foreign Relations and a fellow of the U.K. Royal College of Pathologists, the Royal College of Physicians, the Royal Society of Arts, the Academy of Medical Sciences, and the Royal Society. He is a Commander of the British Empire.

William Rouse, Ph.D., is the Alexander Crombie Humphreys Chair and the director of the Center for Complex Systems and Enterprises at Stevens Institute of Technology. Previously he was a professor in the School of Industrial and Systems Engineering at the Georgia Institute of Technology. He was the chief executive officer of two software companies—Enterprise Support Systems and Search Technology. He has held faculty positions at the University of Illinois, Delft University of Technology, and Tufts University. Among many advisory roles, he has served as a member of the U.S. Air Force Scientific Advisory Board and a member of the Department of Defense Senior Advisory Group on Modeling and Simulation. He has received the Joseph Wohl Outstanding Career Award and the Norbert Wiener Award from the IEEE (Institute of Electrical and Electronics Engineers) Systems, Man, and Cybernetics Society; a Centennial Medal and a Third Millennium Medal from IEEE; and the O. Hugo Schuck Award from the American Automation Control Council. He is a fellow of IEEE, the International Council on Systems Engineering, the Institute for Operations Research and Management Science, and the Human Factors and Ergonomics Society. He is a member of the National Academy of Engineering.

William Stead, M.D., is the chief strategy officer for Vanderbilt University Medical Center, where he also holds appointments as the McKesson Foundation Professor of Biomedical Informatics and Professor of Medicine. He has served as the president of the American College of Medical Informatics and the chair of the board of regents of the National Library of Medicine. He is a founding fellow of the American College of Medical Informatics and the American Institute for Medical and Biological Engineering, and he served as the founding editor-in-chief of the *Journal of the American Medical Informatics Association*. He received his B.A., M.D., and residency training in internal medicine and nephrology from Duke University. His awards include the Collen Award for Excellence in Medical Informatics and the Lindberg Award for Innovation in Informatics. He is the chair of the National Committee on Vital and Health Statistics of the Department of Health and Human Services. He is a member and former councilor of the National Academy of Medicine.

Cornelia Ulrich, Ph.D., is the executive director of the Comprehensive Cancer Center at the Huntsman Cancer Institute and also the Jon M. and Karen Huntsman Presidential Professor in Cancer Research in the Department of Population Health Sciences at The University of Utah. Her research focuses on lifestyle and biologic factors in cancer prevention and cancer prognosis. She is also the principal investigator of the Huntsman Cancer Institute Total Cancer Care Protocol in the ORIEN network of cancer centers. Earlier she was the head of the Department of Preventive Oncology at the German Cancer Research Center and the director of the National Center for Tumor Diseases in Heidelberg, Germany. She has served as a co-chair of the German Society of Epidemiology cancer group and was a guest member of the committee for the implementation of the German Cancer Plan. She serves on numerous national and international advisory boards and leadership committees for groups, including the National Institutes of Health, the International Agency for Research on Cancer, and the American Association for Cancer Research. She is a senior editor for *Cancer Epidemiology, Biomarkers, & Prevention*. She received her M.Sc. from Oregon State University and Ph.D. from the University of Washington. She is a recipient of the American Association of Cancer Research Bristol-Myers Squibb Young Investigator Award, a former Fulbright scholar, and a member of the European Academy of Cancer Sciences.

Staff

Guru Madhavan, Ph.D. (*Study Director*), is the director of programs of the National Academy of Engineering. His portfolio of work at the National Academies of Sciences, Engineering, and Medicine has included leading the analyses for making prescription medicines affordable, directing a global health forum on infectious diseases, and conducting the research, design, and development of a systems analysis platform for prioritizing new vaccines. A systems engineer by background, he received his M.S. and Ph.D. in biomedical engineering and an M.B.A. from the State University of New York. He has served as a technical adviser to the Department of Health and Human Services and has worked in the medical device industry as a research scientist developing cardiac surgical catheters for ablation therapy. He has served as a vice president of the Institute of Electrical and Electronics Engineers (IEEE)-USA and was a founding member of the Global Young Academy. His honors include the

National Academies' Innovator Award, National Academy of Medicine's Cecil Medal, AAMI–Becton Dickinson Award for Professional Achievement, Washington Academy of Sciences' Krupsaw Award for engineering sciences and education, and Professional Achievement Award from the Society of Asian Scientists and Engineers as well as being named a distinguished young scientist by the World Economic Forum. For his books and lectures, he has also received the IEEE-USA Award for Distinguished Literary Contributions Furthering Public Understanding and the Advancement of the Engineering Profession.

Francis Amankwah, M.P.H., is an associate program officer in the Health and Medicine Division of the National Academies of Sciences, Engineering, and Medicine. Earlier, he provided research support for two forums focused on global violence prevention and on public–private partnerships for global health and safety in the National Academies' Board on Global Health. He also served as a research associate for the National Academies' Board on Children, Youth, and Families, where he provided research support for two consensus studies focused on peer victimization and bullying and on fostering school success for English and dual-language learners. For his work at the National Academies, he has received the Mount Everest staff achievement award from the Health and Medicine Division. He earned his M.P.H. and a graduate certificate in global planning and international development from Virginia Tech. He was raised in Ghana and earned his B.S. degree in agricultural science from Kwame Nkrumah University of Science and Technology.

Annalee Gonzales is an administrative assistant with the Board on Health Care Services and the National Cancer Policy Forum at the National Academies of Sciences, Engineering, and Medicine. She previously served as a senior program assistant for two reports from the National Academies on peer victimization and bullying and on fostering school success for English and dual-language learners. Prior to joining the National Academies she worked as an editorial and administrative coordinator at the National Association for Bilingual Education. She earned her B.A. in communication from Trinity University.

Sharyl Nass, Ph.D., serves as the director of the Board on Health Care Services and the director of the National Cancer Policy Forum at the National Academies of Sciences, Engineering, and Medicine. To help enable the best possible care for all patients, the board engages independent, scholarly analysis of the organization, financing, effectiveness, workforce, and delivery of health care, with an emphasis on quality, cost, and accessibility. The National Cancer Policy Forum examines policy issues pertaining to the entire continuum of cancer research and care. For 20 years, Dr. Nass has worked on a broad range of health and science policy topics, including the quality and safety of health care and clinical trials, developing technologies for precision medicine, and strategies for large-scale biomedical science. She received her B.S. and an M.S. from the University of Wisconsin–Madison, completed her Ph.D. at Georgetown University, and conducted postdoctoral research at the Johns Hopkins University School of Medicine and the Max Planck Institute in Germany. She has received the Cecil Medal for Excellence in Health Policy Research, a Distinguished Service Award from the National Academies, and the Institute of Medicine staff team achievement award as a team leader.

Appendix C

Disclosure of Unavoidable Conflict of Interest

The conflict of interest policy of the National Academies of Sciences, Engineering, and Medicine (http://www.nationalacademies.org/coi) prohibits the appointment of an individual to a committee authoring a Consensus Study Report if the individual has a conflict of interest that is relevant to the task to be performed. An exception to this prohibition is permitted if the National Academies determines that the conflict is unavoidable and the conflict is publicly disclosed. A determination of a conflict of interest for an individual is not an assessment of that individual's actual behavior or character or ability to act objectively despite the conflicting interest.

It was determined that George Poste had a conflict of interest in relation to his service on the Committee on a National Strategy for Cancer Control in the United States because he serves on the board of directors of Exelexis, Inc., and Caris Life Sciences.

The National Academies concluded that in order for the committee to accomplish the tasks for which it was established, its membership must include at least one person with current industry experience in drugs, devices, and vaccines development. As described in his biographical summary, Dr. Poste has extensive and current experience in multiple industry sectors that focus on developing preventive, diagnostic, and therapeutic interventions for cancers.

The National Academies determined that the experience and expertise of Dr. Poste was needed for the committee to accomplish the task for which it has been established. The National Academies could not find another available individual with the equivalent experience and expertise who does not have a conflict of interest. Therefore, the National Academies concluded that the conflict was unavoidable and publicly disclosed it through the National Academies Projects and Activities System (https://nationalacademies.org/pa).